The Ultimate Medical Scribe Handbook

Primary Care
3rd Edition

Aaron Thompson;
Kyle Kingsley, MD

DEDICATION

This book is dedicated to all those scribes that seek to further understand medicine before they begin their graduate medical education. Medicine is a long journey and we hope this manual will be the first step in a long and rewarding career in the field.

ACKNOWLEDGMENTS

Thank you to all those who have been an integral part of our training as physicians and scribes, to family and friends, and all others that have contributed directly and indirectly to our being and this publication.

CONTENTS

Section 1: Basics for the Medical Scribe

Section 2: Family Medicine

INTRODUCTION

The following guide is intended as the definitive medical scribe training manual for scribes working in the primary care setting. This manual is designed for new or experienced medical scribes, with little to no prior clinical experience, working for any organization. Any scribe can learn the bare minimum to do their job, but this book is designed to maximize your documentation skills and understanding of clinical medicine. Whether you have no medical experience at all, or you are an experienced scribe looking to increase your abilities, you will find that the focused yet comprehensive materials in this book will improve your knowledge and technical skills as a scribe.

This book can be used in addition to other training materials to help you improve your overall understanding of medicine and performance as a medical scribe. On-the-job training will of course be the major means by which you will learn your facility's workflow, your doctor's preferences, and the navigation of your electronic medical record, but mastering the basics in this book will put you on the fast track to understanding clinical medicine.

Anatomy, medical terminology, and medical knowledge as a whole can only be mastered if you take the time. Learning is not a passive process. Reading this book will be help you recognize medical terms, but if you want to truly memorize new information then you have to make an effort to learn it. No one is perfect and you will make mistakes—learn from them! The mark of great scribes and future doctors is the ability to learn from mistakes, not the absence of making them.

Throughout this handbook, in an attempt to decrease the use of "his/her" on every page, you will notice that we have chosen either the masculine form "him" or even the technically incorrect "they" by default. This is merely for ease of writing and in no way reflects any bias on our part regarding the sex of the practicing physician.

This is the third edition of this book and through our own attempts at teaching new scribes and the successes and failures from doing so, we hope that we too have learned from our mistakes and have made this second edition more meaningful and more applicable to work as a medical scribe. However, we would very much welcome your feedback and suggestions for ways to improve future editions. You can leave us feedback at the email address medicalscribetraining@gmail.com.

If you are interested in more hands-on and interactive learning, we offer online medical scribe training courses including a course specifically designed around this book and primary care practice. You can learn more about the primary care course and our other online courses at www.MedicalScribeTraining.net.

It should, at last, be noted that the ideas in this book are not written in stone. It is vital that as a medical scribe you adapt to the physician with whom you are working. We have tried to straddle the boundary between providing excessive and insufficient amounts of information for the new medical scribe. Sometimes this leads to generalizations that are exactly that—they are true *most* of the time but may not be true *all* of the time. They can be helpful for learning concepts, but you should consult a formal medical resource to learn more.

SECTION 1:

BASICS FOR THE MEDICAL SCRIBE

1. THE MEDICAL SCRIBE

Who Are Scribes?

Medical scribes are the latest addition to the medical team. Although the clinic is our focus here, medical scribes also work in the emergency department, hospital, clinic and urgent care settings. Many scribes are highly motivated college students that are using the job as a stepping stone to medical, physician assistant, or nursing school. Medical assistants, nurses and other clinical or clerical staff have also started to move into a scribe role in some clinics. Universally, scribes are bright, hard-working and excited about medicine.

What Does A Scribe Do?

The main role of the medical scribe is to record—into the medical record—the detailed information from a patient's visit to clinic. It should be noted that the general role and scope of the scribe's job is highly dependent on the physician, physician group, and setting/hospital in which the scribe works.

Documentation

Nearly all medical information at reputable hospitals is now entered into computers and forms part of the electronic medical record (EMR). Medical documentation is important for several reasons. The EMR is the repository where all important information about the patient's medical care is kept. It also serves as a billing tool by which all fees are generated for both the doctor and hospital. In addition, the EMR records a hospital's compliance with core and quality measures, which we will address, in detail, later in this handbook. The EMR may also serve as a defense against legal claims directed at the doctor and/or hospital. For all of these reasons, accurate medical documentation is very important.

Maintenance and generation of the EMR can be quite time consuming and take significant portions of the doctors' time away from patient care. In addition, some physicians are not as "tech-savvy" and are slow to navigate the EMR. The medical information must either be manually typed in, transcribed with voice-recognition software (e.g. Dragon®), or with use of a dictation service in which the physician verbally records a message that is later transcribed into the patient's medical record. Your main job as a scribe is to take the bulk of this task away from the doctors by producing effective documentation that must only be proofread by the physician at the end of the patient encounter or shift. The specifics of documentation will be addressed thoroughly in later chapters.

Patient Flow

After mastering the art of documentation, you can start to contribute more to the patient flow in the clinic. For instance, scribes are able to monitor lab results (telling the doctors when they are available). They can pull up completed x-rays onto viewing screens, enter doctors' x-ray readings into the medical record, and help access old medical records or other information, such as researching a topic or pulling up other academic materials for the physician.

There are also several things a scribe SHOULD NOT DO! Scribes should never make physical contact with patients (other than a possible handshake, if offered). Scribes should not pass medical information between medical professionals (this is not your job). The scribe should never give any medical advice or provide medical care to patients. In fact, scribes are restricted to only a clerical role in conjunction with the physician. Under no circumstances should the scribe enter orders or complete prescriptions. It is also strongly recommended that you never act as a translator in the medical scribe role. This opens you and your scribe provider to significant liability, even if you are a native fluent speaker of the language. We have devoted an entire later section to scribe pitfalls that it is required reading for any medical scribe!

What Are Scribes' Goals?

Scribes come into the job with many goals and expectations. The majority of scribes want to gain experience in the medical field prior to pursuing a career in medicine, nursing or related endeavors. Some scribes are looking to develop a long-term, stimulating career in the scribe industry.

Many scribes find that they gain an extensive, practical foundation of knowledge that will serve them throughout their medical education. Learning the materials in this manual and then applying them in the real world will provide you with a significant jumpstart in your medical documentation and logistic abilities. Some scribes are able to obtain proficiency in medical documentation similar to that of a fourth year medical student or even an intern (1st year in residency). When the rest of your medical or nursing school classmates are learning to write the medical note, the proficient scribe would be able to focus on learning the medicine. Many scribes are also able to outperform their colleagues during clinical rotations as they have a well-developed logistical knowledge within the hospital and have formed relationships with medical providers.

Scribe Ability Checklist

Below is a checklist for general abilities you should strive for as you progress in your training and work as a medical scribe in clinic. This list is by no means exhaustive, but provides a general goal sheet for the motivated student. You should understand, adhere to, and know these topics:

- Electronic medical record navigation
- HIPAA and patient privacy
- Flow and function of the ED
- Basic medical terminology
- General anatomy and physiology
- Methodology of writing an HPI
- Awareness of billing principles as they pertain to the medical note
- Common medications

The Scribe's Unwritten Roles

The medical scribe's role is difficult to define precisely. In addition to the obvious tasks previously outlined, the scribe should do more. The unwritten role is to be assertive, but not too bold in dealing with a physician. You have to figure out how to best help the physician with whom you are working while staying within the scope of your position. You should be quietly competent, not pestering, yet always available if needed. You should always be getting things done without being told (once you learn the job).

The single most important goal for the scribe is to be effective in all you do. Don't just do the minimum; take the next step and master all aspects of your job. Your exact role will be defined by the setting and system in which you work. Be flexible and effective; work hard. It will be noticed.

The Electronic Medical Record (EMR)

The EMR is a system that generates and stores a digital version of patient information and is accessible by clinicians in multiple settings including the emergency room and hospital. The electronic medical record or "EMR" can completely define a scribe's role. It is a repository into which patients' medical notes and information can be entered, saved, and accessed in the future. Another closely related term is the electronic health record or "EHR." Although frequently used interchangeably, the EHR is in theory accessible to all parties involved in the patient's care, including the patient and non-medical personnel. The differences between EMR and EHR are beyond the scope of this book and not important to your work as a medical scribe. We will use the term EMR going forward, but consider that many clinics have systems that would fall into the EHR category.

EMRs vary dramatically in user-friendliness and functionality. Some EMRs are very robust and even helpful to an adept user. Other EMRs are a major hurdle to improved patient care in that they are not user-friendly and consume large portions of provider time just to navigate and enter materials into each record. As a scribe you have no choice but to master the system you are using. Many scribes' abilities with the EMR will even surpass the physicians with whom they work!

HITECH Act and Meaningful Use (MU)

The Health Information Technology for Economic and Clinical Health Act, or HITECH act, was enacted in 2009 by the US department of health and human services. Through this act $25.9 billion in federal funds are being used to promote and expand the "meaningful use" of EHRs throughout the country. Essentially providers and organizations who meet the meaningful use (MU) criteria will initially be given incentives from the CMS, and eventually (2015) there will be penalties for not complying with the MU measures.

The main components of MU include using the EHR for activities such as e-prescribing, electronic order entry, drug allergy checks, recording patient demographics and many others. MU is being rolled out in several stages. To meet the stage one MU measures eligible providers and hospitals must meet all core MU measures (14 for hospitals and 15 for eligible providers) and they must meet 5 of 10 "menu items" a defined percentage of the time.

As a scribe it is important that you have a basic understanding of the HITECH act and MU criteria as it applies to your specific EMR and health care setting.

Training Overview

This handbook is designed as a heads-up primer before you begin hands-on training. This book can be used by itself or in addition to another scribe program's training materials.

Most formal scribe training programs have several components. This is a general outline of things you can expect in most training programs:

1. Didactics: online, classroom or written materials or a combination of all three. Many scribe programs have a qualifying exam prior to moving on to clinical training.
2. Mock patient encounters: this often consists of initial mock patient encounters in an online, video or staged setting.
3. Shadowing: one-on-one training or medical scribe shadowing is a fundamental part of all scribe training programs. A scribe trainee will follow and learn from either a scribe trainer or more experienced scribe.

4. Working independently: often there is some form of "trial period" during or after which the scribe starts working independently with physicians.

5. Performance reviews: frequently medical records on which the scribe has worked will be reviewed and feedback will be given to the scribe.

6. Ongoing professional development: online training modules or other learning is common (such as learning or presenting an "advanced scribe topic" in this book).

2. PRIVACY, HIPAA, AND PROFESSIONALISM

Confidentiality

You will be functioning in a sensitive medical environment as part of the medical team. As members of the medical team we cannot share patient information with anyone who is not part of the medical team without the patient's permission. A good rule of thumb is to keep all particulars of your job/experiences to yourself. Not even the slightest violation of confidentiality will be tolerated in this setting. If ever a patient is uncomfortable with you in the room (such as more sensitive exam area), you will be asked to leave. Generally, all medical scribes are required to go through confidentiality training prior to starting the job.

HIPAA

HIPAA is the acronym commonly used to describe the Health Insurance Portability and Accountability Act. In 1996, this federal legislation created national standards for the privacy and security of patient health information. HIPAA, as well as state privacy laws, creates certain obligations for health care providers and staff, as well as rights for the patients. In general you will be required to go through your organization's HIPAA training prior to starting as a medical scribe.

Here is a brief summary of HIPAA privacy compliance:

- Protected health information (PHI) is any individually identifiable health information (e.g. name, address, birth date, Social Security Number, medical record number).
- HIPAA covers all protected health information, regardless of whether the information is or has been in electronic form.
- PHI may be accessed *without* patient consent when it is done for treatment purposes. In addition, it may be disclosed to other bodies when a person or the public is under an imminent threat to their health and if this disclosure may prevent or lessen the threat.
- Only staff members involved in the treatment of a specific patient are granted access to that patient's medical record; it is an infraction of patient privacy to look at the records of a patient

when you are not part of that patient's care team. This includes the medical records of family members, friends, neighbors, co-workers, etc.

- Limit most disclosures of protected health information to the minimum necessary for the intended purpose.

Professionalism

You are expected to dress, groom and carry yourself in a professional manner at all times. Blue jeans, tee shirts, etc. are not acceptable. Company policies vary, but usually uniforms will be provided for each scribe after his/her probation period. It is expected that you wear your uniform and photo ID badge for every shift. Also, perfumes, strongly scented hairsprays, lotions, etc. are not allowed in the hospital.

Do not address patients unless they address you (except for the obvious hello, excuse me, etc.). Your focus is the documentation, not the patient.

You are expected to be punctual and reliable (ten minutes early is always a good habit). It is your responsibility to notify the proper people as soon as possible if a conflict arises with a shift. If you are able to get someone to take your place/trade with you it is even better.

You must be excessively polite in all your interaction with nurses, doctors, patients and all other staff. Don't take anything personally. You can add to a positive atmosphere in the clinic (and bringing in food to share often helps).

Liability

The physician is responsible for proofreading the documentation you help to provide. You are, however, responsible for your behavior. Any breach of confidentiality or professionalism may result in summary removal from your program.

Pitfalls for the Medical Scribe

There are several common pitfalls for the medical scribe. We will divide these into three general categories: 1) Confidentiality 2) Professional and 3) Social.

Confidentiality Pitfalls

The single greatest pitfall for medical scribes is the violation of one or more confidentiality rules. It is very tempting for scribes to discuss cases with family or friends, but generally it is wise to keep details of your job private. You should never take pictures of anything at work, or text anything while at work. Even the perception of inappropriate behavior can cause significant problems for you. As a rule, you should only talk to the physician(s) with whom you are working about the patients for whom you are currently caring for. It should become second-nature that whenever you do discuss a patient, whether with the physician or other staff members, that you should not include any personal information like their name, date of birth, or medical record number. Referencing a patient by their room number is often the best practice.

You also should never enter a patient's record if you are not involved in the patient's care. It may be tempting to look through the charts for interesting patients, but this is a frank violation of confidentiality policies and absolutely prohibited.

Professional Pitfalls

As a scribe you may be very inclined to offer help when someone asks. For example, a patient sees you in the hall and asks you for help to the bathroom. You help that patient into the bathroom after which they fall and break a hip. It later turns out that the patient was not to be out of the bed in the first place and you are given "credit" with helping the patient to the bathroom. A lawsuit follows and you are named in the lawsuit. **In summary, you are not to provide patient care in any capacity as a scribe!** While this example seems rather obvious, there are many more subtle situations that you must pay attention to avoid working outside the scope of your scribe position.

Other professional pitfalls include documentation errors such as missed information or putting information in the wrong patient's chart/record. If this happens you should immediately notify the physician with whom you are working and explain the situation. You must have absolute integrity with regard to patient documentation.

It is very important that you stay the course and be certain you have done a thorough, complete sign-out prior to leaving clinic. It is expected that you complete a note on each patient you saw with the physician. Any absolutely unavoidable exceptions to this should be communicated to your physician before you leave your shift.

Social Pitfalls

Interpersonal relationship problems are another pitfall for the medical scribe. Your job is not to be involved in office politics; staying "above the fray" is a good general policy. You should be friendly and polite, but you have a very important job and this is not a social hour. Also, it is generally unwise to get involved romantically with coworkers and nursing staff.

3. MEDICAL TERMINOLOGY

To begin this chapter, we will first outline general, whole-body terms and concepts. We will then progress methodically from head to toe, marking important anatomical landmarks as we go, much in the same way that you will document the physical exam on patients. Lastly, we have included common medical abbreviations, prefixes/suffixes, and differentiation between commonly confused terms. It is recommended that you thoroughly understand this section prior to your first shift as a scribe.

We must make one note in regards to abbreviations. They may improve your efficiency and understanding of other medical notes, but due to the ever increasing number of abbreviations used in the medical field, there have been duplicate and obscure uses of abbreviations. For this reason, the current sentiment of the medical community is to promote the use of fewer abbreviations so as to avoid confusion. As such, despite the advantages of saved time and space, the use of abbreviations should be limited to the most commonly known terms and conditions. This is true for the terms in this chapter and throughout this book.

General Anatomy and Kinesiology Terms

Anatomy and kinesiology are the study of the human body and movement and terms in this field are vital in medical practice. We will start this section with a few simple anatomy and kinesiology concepts that are generally not known to the layperson.

Proximal means closer to the origin (starting point) of an extremity. In contrast, **distal** means farther out from "the start" of the arm, or leg, or finger/toe. These are common terms used by physicians in all settings. For example, the foot is distal to the knee, the shoulder is proximal to the elbow, and the wrist is distal to the elbow. This is a universally applicable concept and essential for you to understand.

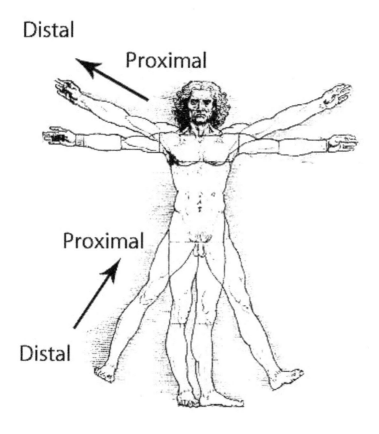

Figure 1: Vitruvian Man, Leonardo da Vinci, circa 1487

Another important concept is medial versus lateral. **Medial** means closer to the midline of the body and **lateral** means farther from the midline. These terms can be absolute or relative. For example, the medial ankle is the inside part of the ankle (closer to the imaginary midline of the body, as illustrated below). Or a finding can be medial or lateral to an anatomical structure (e.g. a laceration just lateral to the left eyebrow). Medial and lateral can generally be applied to any part of the body including the finger, foot, leg, head, chest—essentially everywhere! In the diagram on the right below, medial and lateral are outlined on the patient's right lower extremity.

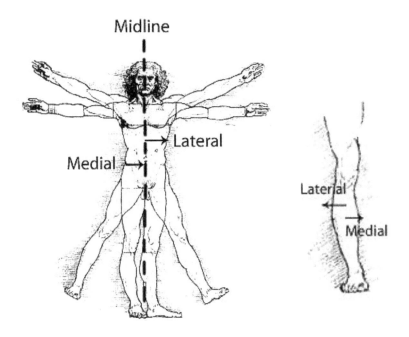

Figure 2: Vitruvian Man – medial vs. lateral

Next is cephalad vs. caudad. **Cephalad** means closer to the head; **caudad** is in the opposite direction ("cauda" technically means "tail" in Latin). Although less commonly used, these are still important terms. Two more important terms are anterior and posterior (not illustrated here). **Anterior** means toward the front of the body (or body part) and **posterior** is toward the back.

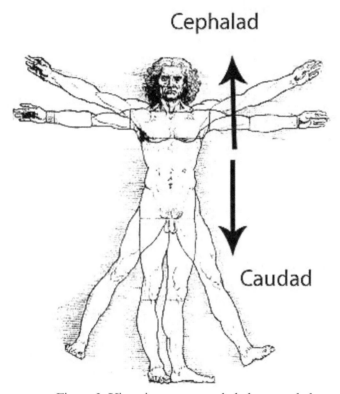

Figure 3: Vitruvian man – cephalad vs. caudad

Adduction is movement of an extremity toward the midline. **Abduction** is movement away from the midline. A good way to remember this is aDduction (as in aDdition) is TOWARD the midline and aBduction is away from the midline.

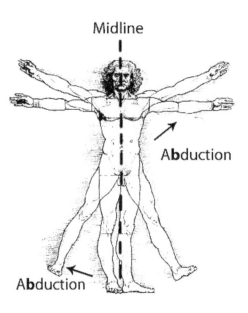

Figures 4 and 5: Vitruvian man – abduction and adduction

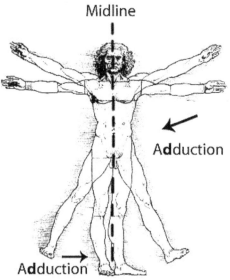

Summary of Key Anatomical Descriptors

Abduction	bring away from the midline of the body
Adduction	bring toward the midline of the body
Anterior	front of the body
Caudad	towards the "tail," or the opposite of cephalad
Cephalad	closer to the head
Distal	away or further from the origin of an appendage (e.g. the ulna is distal to the humerus)
Dorsal	toward the back (including back of the hand or top of the feet)
Lateral	away from the midline of the body
Medial	toward the midline of the body
Posterior	back of the body
Prone position	lying face down
Proximal	closer to the origin of an appendage (e.g. the humerus is proximal to the ulna)
Supine position	lying on the back

Descriptions of the Hands

Dorsal	back side of the hand
Palmar	palm side
Volar	palm side

Descriptions of the Feet

Dorsal	top of the foot
Plantar	sole of the foot
Volar	sole of the foot

Basic Human Anatomy

The typical adult has 214 bones in the human body. Most of these are unnecessary for you to know (at least at this point in your medical career), but there are several bones and articulations (a.k.a. joints) that you should know as a scribe. The following section will provide an overview of the major bones and joints that are essential to your knowledge. Many of these anatomical terms serve as valuable landmarks for describing the location of a patient's pain or injury, but we attempted to provide a few examples of specific abnormalities too.

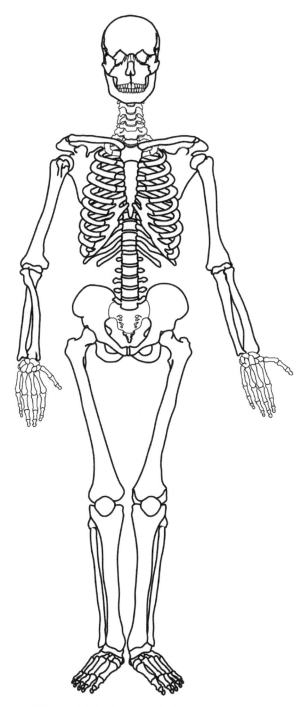

Figure 6: The human skeleton

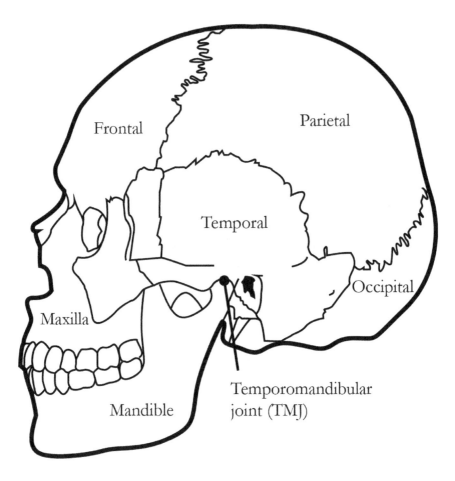

Figure 7: The cranial and facial bones

There are four major cranial regions that overlie the four major cranial bones. The four bones are labeled in Figure 7 and include the:

- Frontal bone – this single bone makes up the forehead

- Parietal bones – these two symmetric bones lie on either side of the sagittal suture (i.e. the midline of the skull)

- Temporal bones – the temporal bones form the bony areas around each ear (which can be seen by the opening in the skull in this region) and comprises part of the skull base. The carotid arteries, vestibulocochlear complex (balance and hearing centers), and several facial nerves are protected by this region. A fracture in this region may cause dizziness, hearing loss or facial paralysis. Hemotympanum (blood in the middle ear) is a sign of a temporal bone fracture

- Occipital bone – this single bone forms the posterior of the skull. It is a common region for head trauma after falling backwards and is also a common region for pain during a migraine headache

The two facial bones that are also important include the:

- Maxillary bones (singular maxilla, plural maxillae) – these two bones comprise the upper jaw. The upper teeth (#1-16) are embedded in the maxilla.

- Mandible – the lower jaw or mandible is the large bone that hinges at the temporal bone.

The primary joint that you need to know is the:

- Temporomandibular joint (TMJ) – the articulation of the mandible and temporal bone, connected by ligaments that stretch and allow the jaw to open and close.

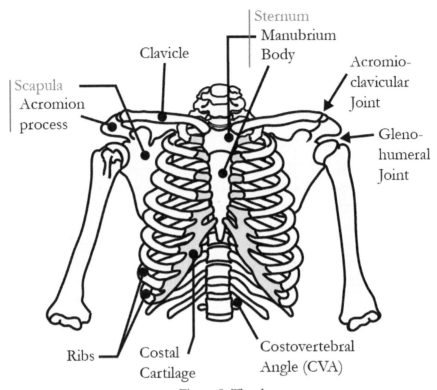

Figure 8: The thorax

The bones of the thorax protect vital body organs (heart, lungs, liver, kidneys, etc.). Minor trauma may cause a bony injury (fracture or dislocation) while major trauma may result in damage to the internal organs. You will most frequently encounter the terminology during the physical exam as the physician describes abnormal findings (e.g. the patient is exquisitely tender over the right AC joint). The bones are labeled on the right side of the pictured skeleton (your left) and the major articulations are labeled on the opposite side with arrows.

- Scapula – also known as the shoulder blade, the scapulae form the flat bone on each side the upper back. It forms the basic "socket" (the glenoid fossa) that makes up the ball and socket joint of the shoulder.
  - Acromion – an appendage of the scapula, the acromion process extends anteriorly and articulates with the clavicles, forming the acromioclavicular (AC) joint

- Clavicles – these two bones connect medially to the sternum and laterally to the acromion process, forming the AC joint.

- Humerus – the upper arm bone that articulates with the scapula to form the shoulder

- Ribs – there are 12 thoracic ribs (corresponding to the 12 thoracic vertebrae), 10 of which connect the vertebral column to the sternum and form the protective cavity for the heart and lungs. The remaining 2 are called "floating ribs" and do not connect to the sternum

- Sternum – the sternum is actually made of three bones including the manubrium (the top part), the body (the middle), and the xyphoid process (the small point at the bottom). It connects to the clavicles superiorly (at the clavicular notches) and to the ribs laterally via the costal cartilage

- Costal cartilage and the costochondral junction– this is the region where the ribs connect to the sternum via a short piece of cartilage ("chondral" refers to cartilage, and "costal" to the ribs). This area may become inflamed and painful, a condition caused costochondritis

The major articulations of the thorax include the:

- Costovertebral angle (CVA) – the angle formed by the junction of the vertebrae with the lower ribs (in the mid-back). This is an important region as each kidney lies partly below the CVA and palpation or percussion of this region may result in pain in the case of acute pyelonephritis (a "kidney infection"). Note that although we grouped this with the articulations, it is actually more of an anatomical landmark than a true articulation

- Acromioclavicular (AC) joint – the connection of the clavicle to the anterior process of the scapula. This joint may become dislocated due to blunt trauma of the shoulder

- Glenohumeral joint – the ball and socket joint formed by the head of the humerus and glenoid fossa of the scapula. This is the technical term for the shoulder joint

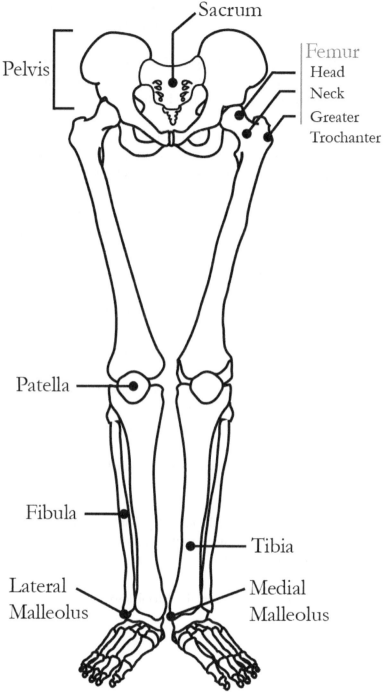

Figure 9: The lower extremities

The bones of the pelvis and lower extremities are large and fairly easy to remember. The most important bones include the:

- Sacrum – the fused bony region that connects the lumbar vertebrae to the coccyx (a.k.a. the tailbone, the small pointy structure at the bottom of the sacrum) as well as the two hip bones to each other

- Pelvis – the pelvis is the collective structure formed by the fusion of the sacrum and the two "hip" bones (that are actually made of three smaller bones called the ilium, ischium, and pubis)

- Femur – the large bones the run the length of the thigh and connect superiorly to the pelvis and inferiorly to the tibia (and patella). A hip fracture is the colloquial term for a proximal femur fracture, which typically occurs at the neck of the femur
  - Femoral head – the "ball" that forms the ball and socket of the hip joint by connecting to the acetabulum (the "socket" in the hip)
  - Femoral neck – this is the common place to sustain a hip fracture
  - Greater trochanter – the large, palpable bony protrusion on the lateral femur. Trochanteric bursitis is not uncommon to see in clinic (see "bursitis" on page 113)

- Patella – the floating bone that is embedded in the patellar tendon and forms the kneecap

- Tibia – the large bone in the lower leg that bears nearly all of the weight of the lower leg. It connects to the femur to form the knee joint and to the foot to form the ankle.

- Fibula – the small bone in the lateral lower leg that bears very little weight

The major joints of the lower extremities include the:

- Hip joint – a ball and socket joint formed by the socket of the hip called the acetabulum and the femoral head

- Knee joint – the joint connecting the femur to the tibia. There are several soft tissues within the knee that are quite complex and are unnecessary for our knowledge (the collateral ligaments, menisci, bursa, patellar tendon, etc.)

- Malleoli – the large bony protrusions on the medial and lateral aspect of each ankle are formed by the ends of the tibia and fibula, respectively. These are called the medal and lateral malleoli (singular malleolus) and are the most important landmarks of each ankle.

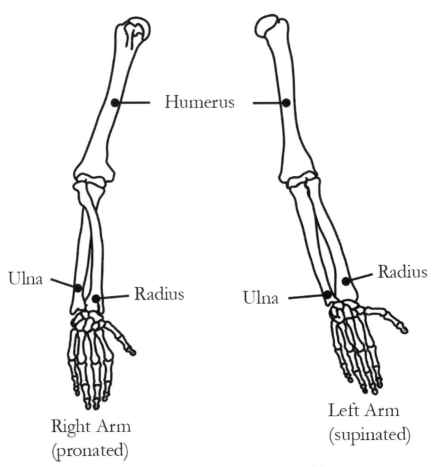

Figure 10: Bones of the upper extremities

The bones of the upper extremities are very similar to the legs in that there is one large bone in the upper arm and two smaller bones in the lower arm. The forearm bones (radius and ulna) are somewhat more troublesome because they rotate around each other with supination/pronation. This means that what is the medial forearm when the hand is supinated (ulnar aspect) is different than the medial forearm when the hand is pronated (radial aspect). Thus, it is less common to describe something as "over the medial forearm" because people (including doctors) forget which way the hand is turned during proper anatomical descriptions (supinated is technically correct). Instead, the radius and ulna are used as landmarks when describing the location of something on the forearm. For example, saying there is "a laceration over the radial aspect of the distal forearm" would be common. Each of the bones, in more detail, are the:

-Humerus – the upper arm bone that connects with the scapula to form the shoulder joint. Inferiorly, it forms the elbow joint where it connects with the radius and ulna

-Radius – the forearm bone that is straight when the forearm is supinated (left arm), but rotates around the ulna with pronation of the forearm (right arm). The radius connects the elbow to the wrist at the thumb side of the hand; that is why the radial pulse can be felt just proximal to the wrist on the thumb side of the forearm.

-Ulna – the forearm bone that connects the "pinky" side of the wrist to the elbow. The ulna forms the major connection to the humerus and thus the elbow joint.

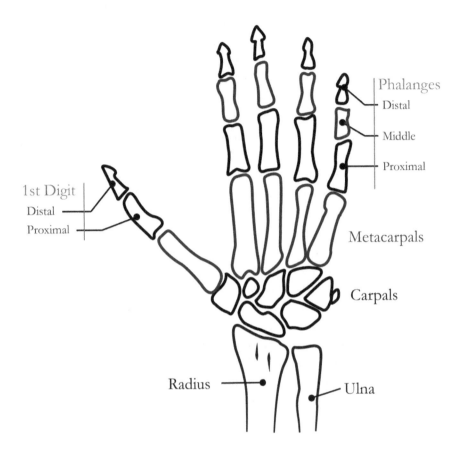

Figure 11: Bones of the wrist and hand

The bones of the hand are important landmarks for injuries that occur to the wrist, hand and fingers. The fingers may be described with lay person terms (like index, middle, ring or pinky finger) or by more technical terms. Technical descriptions of the fingers most commonly use the number system, in which the thumb is the 1st finger (or first digit), and the pinky is the 5th digit.

-Radius - as already covered in Figure 10, the radius and ulna are the bones of the forearm that articulate with the carpal bones to form the wrist joint—the radius joining on the thumb side

-Ulna – the forearm bone on the pinky side of the wrist

-Carpal bones – there are technically 10 separate carpal bones, but for our purposes it is unnecessary to known the names and locations of each; they are often poor landmarks because you cannot easily feel or see the separations between them

-Metacarpals – the bones in each digit that make up the body of the hand

-Phalanges – the three individual bones in each finger (except for the thumb, which only has two bones). They are known as the proximal, middle, and distal phalanges (*singular phalanx*)

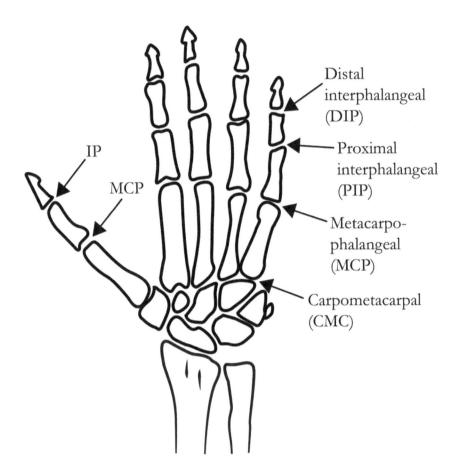

Figure 12: Articulations of the hand

The joints of the hand are maybe more important than knowing the individual bones of the hand. These joints are very easy landmarks to use when describing various injuries of the hand and the terms below you will likely encounter on a regular basis.

-Carpometacarpal (CMC) joint – the joint created by the joining of the carpals to the metacarpals; it is far more common to hear CMC joint rather than the full name for the term

-Metacarpophalangeal (MCP) joint – the joint made by the connection of the metacarpals to the proximal phalanges. This joint forms what are typically called the "knuckles"

-Proximal interphalangeal joint (PIP) – this is the first of two joints that are formed by the 3 phalanges in each finger. This is good landmark for describing injuries of the fingers. For example, a laceration may be described as "just distal to the 2nd PIP joint," which would mean the patient has a laceration overlying the middle phalanx of the index finger

-Distal interphalangeal joint (DIP) – this is the second of two joints formed by the 3 phalanges in each finger. Just like the PIP joint, the DIP joint is a common landmark when describing finger injuries

The thumb, unlike the other four digits, only has two phalanges. Thus, instead of having 2 separate joints (the PIP and DIP), it only has one interphalangeal joint. As you will see, the great toe (a.k.a. the big toe) has a very similar structure.

-Interphalangeal (IP) joint – the single joint in the thumb

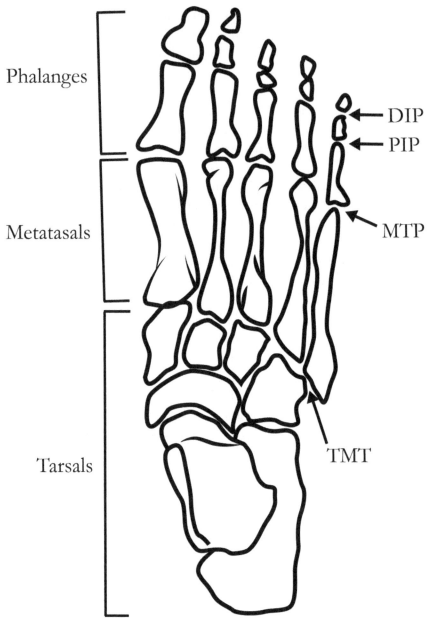

Phalanges

DIP

PIP

Metatasals

MTP

Tarsals

TMT

Figure 13: Bones and articulations of the foot

The foot is organized in nearly the same fashion as the hand. The major groups of bones include the:

-Tarsal bones – the tarsal bones are similar to the carpals and compose the body of the foot. You do not have to know the names of individual bones (though you're always welcome to do so)

-Metatarsals – the metatarsals compose the distal half of the foot body, but before the toes. The tendons overlying the metatarsals are highly visible and can help you estimate the location of the underlying bones

-Phalanges – the toes are nearly identical in structure to the fingers. Note that like the thumb, the big toe (or great toe) is only made up of two bones, rather than three bones (proximal, middle, distal) like the rest of the toes

The joints connecting the bones of the feet occur in the same general anatomic location as the joints of the hands and are named very similarly. The tarsometatarsal (TMT) joint, metatarsophalangeal (MTP), and the two interphalangeal joints (proximal interphalangeal, distal interphalangeal) are again very important landmarks for describing pain, swelling, redness, etc. that occurs in the feet. For example, gout typically causes pain and redness in the 1st MTP joint (the "knuckle" of the big toe).

Common Abbreviations

ABX	antibiotics	NAD	no acute disease/ no acute distress (contextual)
A&O	alert and oriented		
ASA	aspirin		
BID	twice daily	NPO	nothing by mouth
BM	bowel movement	NS	normal saline
BS	bowel sounds	N/V	nausea/vomiting
C/o	complains of	PERRL	pupils equals, round and reactive to light
CP	chest pain		
CTA	clear to auscultation	PO	*per os* (passed orally)
C/w	consistent with	PRN	as needed
D/C	discharge	PTA	prior to arrival / admission
Ddx	differential diagnosis		
D/T	due to	QD	every day
Dx	diagnosis	QID	four times daily
EBL	estimated blood loss (from surgery)	ROM	range of motion
		RRR	regular rate and rhythm
EMS	emergency medical service	SL	sublingual
EtOH	alcohol	S/P	status post (surgical)
F/C	fever/chills	Sx	symptoms
Fx	fracture	SOB	shortness of breath
GxPy	gravida para (pregnancy)	TID	three times daily
		TM	tympanic membrane
HA	headache	TTP	tenderness to palpation
H/o	history of	UTD	up-to-date
Hx	history	VSS	vital signs stable
IM	intramuscular	WNL	within normal limits
IV	intravenous	yo	years old
IVF	IV fluids		
JVD	jugular venous distention		
LAD	lymphadenopathy		
LOC	loss of consciousness		
MOI	mechanism of injury		
MVA	motor vehicle accident		

Useful Prefixes / Suffixes

General Prefixes

A-   negative or not
Dys-   abnormal
Hyper-   over, greater than
Hypo-   under, less than
Infra-   below
Inter-   between
Intra-   within
Ipsi-   same (e.g. ipsilateral = same side)
Oligo-   a few, a little
Para-   alongside or beside (e.g. paraspinous muscles)
Peri-   around (e.g. periorbital region)
Poly-   many
Sub-   beneath
Super-   in excess, above
Supra-   above
Trans-   situated across or through

Physiological/Pathological Prefixes

Adeno-   relating to a gland
Angio-   blood vessel
Carcino-   cancer
Chol(e)-   pertaining to bile
Cholecyst-   pertaining to the gallbladder
Chondro-   cartilage
Cutane-   skin
Cyst-   pertaining to the urinary bladder (note, see ovarian cyst)
Dys-   bad, difficult
Gastro-   stomach
Gnath-   jaw
Hemat-/Hem-   blood
Hepat-   liver
Myc-   fungus
Nephro-   pertaining to the kidney
Pyelo-   pelvis

Rhin(o)-	nose
Tachy-	fast
Tetan-	rigid, tense
Viscer-	pertaining to the internal organs

Physiological/Pathological Suffixes

—algia	pain
—cardia	heart
—crine	to secrete
—ectomy	surgical removal
—emia	blood
—itis	inflammation
—iasis	condition
—ism	condition
—lith	stone
—odyn	pain
—oma	tumor, mass
—osis	condition
—otomy	surgical incision
—penia	deficiency (e.g. leukopenia)
—pepsia	related to digestion
—pnea	breathing
—pneumo	pertaining to the lungs
—uria	urine

Tricky Vocabulary Pairs

Nauseous/Nauseated

Nauseous means something causes nausea. Nauseated is to have nausea. A patient is nauseated, not nauseous. This is a near universal error in medicine.

Naris/Nares

The medical term for one nostril is naris. The plural of naris is nares. A common error made in medicine is to make the singular of nares "nare," which is not a word.

Dysphagia/Dysphasia

Dysphagia refers to difficulty swallowing; dysphasia is a loss of or deficiency in the ability to use or understand language. You can remember that dysphaGIa is related to the GI system.

Stridorous vs. stridulous/stridulant

Stridorous is a common way to state that a patient has stridor, or noise generated in the upper airway/throat when breathing. Although technically the word that should be used is stridulant or stridulous, stridorous is still frequently used by physicians. We would recommend following your physician's lead on this one.

Oriented/Orientated

These two terms are interchangeable and equivalent, although many try to say that orientated is not correct.

Infection/Inflammation

Infection is the invasion of host tissue by disease-causing organisms such as bacteria. Inflammation is a complex tissue response (red, swollen, painful, "angry-looking") to some stimuli. Infections are one of the many things that can cause inflammation.

Sprain/Strain

These are not the same! A sprain refers to the injury of a ligament. A strain is an injury to tendons or muscles. Remember that the word strain contains the letter "t" as does tendon, and tendons are attached to muscles.

Oral/Aural
Oral has to do with the mouth. Aural is pronounced the same and has to do with hearing.

Follow Up vs. Followup/Follow-up
When used as a verb, the two word form is used. When used as a noun or adjective, followup or follow-up can be used. Examples: "The patient will follow up with Dr. Smith tomorrow." "Followup was arranged for the patient." "Please schedule a follow-up appointment."

Palpitation/Palpation
Palpitation is the sense of an irregular heartbeat or fluttering in the chest. Palpation is feeling something with your hands.

Peritoneal/Perineal/Peroneal
Peritoneal refers to the peritoneum or the lining of the internal organs of the abdomen. Perineal refers to the perineum or the area between the anus and genitals. Peroneal refers to the outer parts of the lower leg, the fibular aspect of the lower leg.

Prostate/Prostrate
The prostate is a gland in the male anatomy. Prostrate is defined as lying face-down in extreme exhaustion or incapacitation. Do not mix up this one! Many patients state they have "prostrate" problems. Know that they are using the wrong word!

Neurologist/Neurosurgeon
The neurologist is responsible for non-surgical nerve and central nervous system issues such as seizures, headaches, and some strokes. Neurosurgeons work with trauma to the head and spinal cord, brain tumors and intracerebral hemorrhage.

4. THE MEDICAL NOTE

The creation of medical notes is a major function of the medical scribe in the clinic. You will become skilled at quickly putting together notes based on the interaction you observe between the doctor and the patient. Some scribes will choose to do notes as the doctor is interviewing the patient using portable computers. Others may choose to quickly jot down notes on paper, and later, when time permits, transcribe the note into the electronic medical record. Some scribes, even when computers are available, keep paper on-hand to document certain parts of the patient encounter because of the lag in maneuvering through the electronic medical record. In any case, the final product (the medical note) is often structured as outlined in the following sections. Different EMRs have cosmetic differences, but the general layout is generally quite similar to the format shown in this chapter.

The SOAP Note

It is important that you first learn the structure of the medical note in its purest form before seeing it used in practice (usually within an electronic medical record). The general form of almost all medical notes is the "SOAP format." This stands for Subjective, Objective, Assessment and Plan. This is the general order in which things are placed in most medical notes.

Subjective: The subjective section is based on information that the patient tells the provider—the patient therefore being deemed "subjective." The chief complaint and history of present illness fall into this category. Review of systems, past medical history, social history, medications, allergies and family history would also likely fall under this category, although these could be considered slightly more objective because they can be more easily verified.

Objective: The objective section is based on information discovered by the physician, who is deemed an objective, unbiased evaluator of the patient. This section includes physical exam findings, labs, and radiology results.

Assessment: What does the physician think is going on? What is the patient's situation? Because the primary care physician may evaluate multiple complaints per visit, each condition evaluated may be given a sentence of two as: "Diabetes mellitus, type II: his A1C today is 7.7. No evidence of neuropathy or nephropathy."

Plan: What is the general treatment plan? Is the patient going to receive any medications? When will they follow up in clinic next? Occasionally, a patient may be directly admitted to the hospital, though this is fairly rare. Continuing with our diabetic male patient, this last step may be written as, "Continue glipizide as he has responded well at this point. Follow-up in 3 months for recheck."

A full clinic note is often formed in the order below. Some very brief notes may not include all of the sections below, as it may "over bill" for the amount of work performed and may obscure the important details from the visit. Following this page, we break down each individual section of the SOAP note. Note that the SOAP headings may not be placed in the note— they are just here to help you understand the general organization of the note.

SUBJECTIVE
Chief Complaint (CC)
History of Present Illness (HPI)
Review of Systems (ROS)
Allergies
Medications
Past Medical History (PMH)
Past Surgical History (PSH)
Family History (FH)
Social History (SH)

OBJECTIVE
Physical Exam (PE)
Laboratory Results
Imaging Results

ASSESSMENT
Diagnosis/Impression
Problem List

PLAN
Medications/Treatment
Follow up

Chief Complaint

The chief complaint, often abbreviated CC, is a brief one (or few) word explanation for why the patient is coming into clinic. Medication follow ups, recent hospitalization follow ups, annual physical exams, sports physicals and well child checks are common examples. Generally speaking this should be the complaint as stated by the patient, not a diagnosis (e.g. shortness of breath is the chief complaint, the diagnosis is pneumonia, and not vice versa). The chief complaint should be quick. Don't dwell on this; spend your time on the HPI.

Some electronic medical records automatically generate the chief complaint, or it may be entered by nursing personnel before you ever see the patient.

Here is a list of some of the most common chief complaints for non-follow up related clinic visits:

- Abdominal discomfort
- Cough
- Diarrhea
- Fever
- High blood pressure
- Shortness of breath
- Urinary frequency / urgency

History of Present Illness (HPI)

The HPI is a concise narrative of the patient's story, usually given by the patient. You will derive this from the questions asked by the doctor and the answers given by the patient. Formatting these details into a single or multiple paragraphs will take time to learn, but it will serve you throughout your medical career. In the following pages we will outline the basic details within and the methodology of writing an HPI.

A good deal of historical information can also be obtained from the patient's electronic medical record (in addition to what the patient tells the physician). The most helpful areas to review while writing an HPI are the past medical history, problem list, and chart review. The past medical history and problem list are very similar and will list the patient's historical conditions and current conditions, respectively, with comments about each one (e.g. diabetes type II – diet controlled, last HgA1C 6.7). The chart review, which will include notes from previous ER, hospital and clinic visits within the same electronic medical record system (e.g. Epic), is probably the most informative place to learn about recent clinic and/or hospital visits (rather than from the patient). It is important that you review these documents and in time—after reading more and more medical notes—you will learn to pick up the pertinent details and summarize them in your own HPIs. This is of supreme importance for follow-up visits (hospital follow-up, medication follow-up, hypertension follow-up, etc.). Hopefully, you will have a better understanding of pertinent details from these notes after reading future chapters.

In some cases, the HPI comes from a source other than the patient. Sometimes a family member or an interpreter intermediate may provide the information for the HPI and it is recommended that you record who provides the history for the HPI, often in the first line of or above the HPI. For example: "The history was obtained from the patient's wife as the patient is non-verbal at this time" or "the history was obtained from the patient using a Spanish interpreter." This information can be added before the HPI as a simple stand-alone sentence. Some electronic medical records will have an area to note from whom the history was obtained. Often limitations to history may also be noted, such as "History limited due to patient dementia." Alternatively, the clinician may note "The patient is deemed a reliable historian." However, using this phrase is less common because it is assumed that the patient is a reasonably reliable historian if not otherwise mentioned.

Your job as a scribe is not to copy questions and the associated answers, but to reorganize and synthesize information into a more coherent HPI. Some doctors will have a more rigid protocol for how they interview patients; others will have more chaotic, random patterns. Regardless of the doctor's style, your HPI should contain the information from each question asked by the physician. Because of the pace with which many physicians ask questions, you will need to develop your own medical shorthand so you can keep up with the conversation without missing important information.

We will detail the common structure of the HPI in the following pages, but to give you a sense of the final product, here is a sample HPI for a regular follow-up visit:

"John is a well-known patient that comes in today for a 6 month follow up. He has been monitoring his blood pressure and brought in a list of measurements since his last visit (average of ~140/85).

He still feels that he has the "beta blocker blues." He feels lethargic. Is sleeping ok. Denies crying or moodiness. He used to be a morning go-getter and now feels very lethargic in the morning. His job of 3 years was also eliminated 1 month ago and so he is now unemployed. He and his wife do not have children but care deeply for their pets and they will likely need to put down their nearly blind horse that is only 8 years old.

His weight is down a few lbs since last visit and he is now ebullient that he can fit into his tuxedo pants from 23 years ago.

He also has some rhinorrhea and post-nasal drip that irritates his stomach and is taking Tums. Zyrtec has not helped."

Writing the HPI

The structure of clinic notes is generally less formulaic and more chaotic than notes in other settings. This is because the doctor may ask questions about the patient's health as a whole (physical, mental, social), which often causes the HPI to wander from topic to topic. It will also be less focused than, say, an ER note where the physician is generally only focused on the chief complaint. Nonetheless we will try to prepare you to write a coherent HPI of your own by the end of this chapter.

We will detail the common structure of the HPI in the following pages, but here is another example of an HPI from a primary care visit:

> "Jane is a typically healthy 18 yo that will be heading to college (U of M) this fall and comes in for a sports physical (swimming). Documents from her pediatrician have not yet been transferred over. She reportedly has a history of recurrent sinusitis and has had 2 surgeries to correct this but still has occasional symptoms.
>
> Her periods have been regular, which began the summer after 6th grade. She has a good friend group and will be rooming with a swimming friend at school. She sees dentistry 2 x per year. Weight has been stable. She eats a varied diet but only drinks chocolate milk once daily and no other regular sources of calcium.
>
> There was a year-long period where she had consistently elevated blood pressure and was seen by cardiology and an allergist and it seemed to resolve on its own."

Step 1: The First Sentence

Typically, the first sentence of an HPI includes the patient's name, age, gender, any pertinent medical history and then their chief complaint. It should provide just enough information to act as a topic sentence without providing too much detail:

> "_Name_ is a _age_ y.o. _gender_ with a history of _past medical history_ who presents with _chief complaint_..."

In clinic, patients may be presenting for an annual physical exam, a sports physical, or a particular complaint. This can be fairly simple and stated plainly, such as:

"John is a typically healthy 18 yo that comes in for a sports physical prior to starting fall football practice."

"John is a typically healthy 18 yo that presents for evaluation of left ankle pain."

This is the simplest first sentence, but it is possible to write much more helpful and informational introductions to the HPI. Like writing a typical essay, the first sentence should act as a topic sentence, introducing you to the basic idea of what is to come later in the paragraph. This should generally include a few basic pieces of contextual information, such as pertinent medical history and one or two words describing the chief complaint.

The First Sentence: Pertinent Medical History

For patients presenting because of a specific complaint, like chest pain, it is important that you include any pertinent medical history in the first sentence of the HPI. This provides context for the chief complaint and will set the tone for much of what is written in the remainder of the HPI. In some cases this will require a basic knowledge of some of the risk factors for various conditions, which you will learn about in later chapters. However, for now, we will address some very straightforward examples. First, consider a typically healthy patient that is presenting with left sided abdominal pain and has a history of (painful) ovarian cysts. Because this past medical history is quite important in discerning the most likely cause of her pain, it is recommended that you mention it in the first sentence and then provide greater detail near the end of the HPI regarding it, if necessary. For example:

"Money Penny is a 33 y.o. female with history of ovarian cysts who presents with left lower quadrant abdominal pain.

(near the end)... "Her last known ovarian cyst was 2 years ago at which time she was seen in the ED and prescribed Norco for pain."

As another example, consider a patient presenting for chest pain. What potential risk factors for heart disease can you list off the top of your head? Some of them are highly publicized and some are more subtle, but they include high blood pressure, high cholesterol, diabetes, smoking and a family history of heart disease. If a patient presenting with chest pain has one or more of these risk factors—or even known coronary artery disease—then this/these should be noted in the first sentence. For this example it would appear as follows:

"John Doe is a 52 y.o. male with a history of hypertension and hyperlipidemia who presents with left sided chest pain..."

Make sense? With those few words we have set the stage for what might be chest pain that is concerning for underlying cardiovascular disease. This lets other readers understand the context of the chief complaint and will stay with them as they read the rest of the HPI, which may be directed towards other cardiovascular signs or symptoms depending on the provider's interaction with the patient—and which you have little control over as a scribe.

Since many clinic visits are not centered on a chief complaint, the structure of the first sentence may vary. However, it should still act as a topic sentence and give the reader a general overview of the patient's reason for presentation and any relevant past medical history. We will provide an example of a follow-up visit HPI in the following section.

The First Sentence: Frequency and/or Location

We recommend that the first sentence of the HPI be kept short and succinct yet still include pertinent past medical history (as mentioned above) and one or two descriptors of the patient's chief complaint. The best descriptor is often simply the location of a patient's pain. Instead of writing that a patient presents with chest pain, specifying that they present with right sided, left sided, or substernal chest pain can be very helpful in framing the focus of the HPI. For example, left sided chest pain tends to be concerning for a myocardial infarction (heart attack), right sided pain may represent pneumonia or a pulmonary embolism, and substernal chest pain may indicate heartburn or costochondritis. So briefly describing the location of patient's pain in the first sentence can go a long way in foreshadowing information in the later parts of your HPI. This is where your basic anatomy may be helpful. However, remember that you always describe the location of a patient's symptoms based upon external landmarks, often based on bony structures. For example, you should never write that a patient presents with "stomach pain" because the stomach is an internal organ. Instead, you would use the term abdominal pain or even epigastric pain. As another example, in a patient with a headache, you would not write that they have "frontal lobe pain"—using the word "lobe" refers to the brain and you should instead write "frontal pain," which refers to the frontal scalp. In the case that a patient has more vague symptoms, the list below may provide a few options to use as a descriptor in the first sentence of your HPI:

Diffuse   Pain does not occur in a specific area but is "all over." For example, a patient may have diffuse abdominal pain, which would be in contrast to epigastric pain (localized to the epigastric region). Synonymous with generalized.

Focal   Occurring in a small, definable region. Synonymous with localized.

Generalized   See diffuse. Generalized abdominal pain is synonymous with diffuse abdominal pain.

Localized   See focal.

As a second descriptor, or in the case that describing the location of symptoms isn't describable (in patients with altered mental status, for example), then describing the frequency of a patient's symptoms can be helpful. Frequency—called "timing" in the OPQRSTA mnemonic discussed later—may answer questions like: Are symptoms constant? Do they come-and-go (a.k.a. intermittent)? Are there certain triggers that induce symptoms, such as exercise or changes in body position?

For example, in a patient with chest pain, rather than just saying "…who presents with left sided chest pain" you could further characterize it by saying that "…who presents with *episodic* left sided chest pain." Some of these words are important in suggesting the cause of a patient's problems. For example, *exertional* chest pain is concerning for a heart condition whereas *pleuritic* chest pain (worse with deep breaths) may represent a pulmonary embolism. And *constant* right lower quadrant pain is suggestive of appendicitis whereas *waxing and waning* pain is more suggestive of a kidney stone. The OPQRST mnemonic discussed later addresses several of these descriptors, but it is often good to provide a single key word early in the HPI and then provide greater detail later (when mentioning the other OPQRST components). A list of words that can be used to help you characterize the frequency of symptoms is given below:

Acute	of short duration or high severity. Symptoms may be "acute on chronic," which is an acute exacerbation of a chronic condition (e.g. lumbar back pain or COPD exacerbations).
Constant	always present
Chronic	over a long duration (months – years) without complete resolution
Episodic	comes in episodes with a defined beginning and end; similar to intermittent
Exertional	presents with some degree of exercise
Intermittent	occurs off-and-on
Persistent	ongoing, consistent; generally refers to a shorter time period than chronic symptoms.
Positional	affected by the position of the body (e.g. standing, sitting, lying down, etc.)
Recurrent	symptoms or condition appear, resolve, and then reappear in a chronic fashion but are generally not chronic conditions. Pneumonia is a good example of this as an infection occurs, resolves with antibiotics, and then returns due to inherent susceptibility or exposure. In contrast, COPD may have acute exacerbations, but the underlying

disorder for the symptoms (anatomical changes) is always present; however, the difference between these terms is not set-in-stone.

Waxing and waning	symptoms fluctuate in severity but remain continually present

In summary, providing these two contextual details (pertinent medical history and one or two descriptors) in the first sentence is highly recommended as these details will provide the context that readers (i.e. physicians) will appreciate as they read the remainder of the HPI. However, be careful not to add too many details in the first sentence; save it for the body of the HPI. As a recap, here is what we have written right now:

"John Doe is a 52 y.o. male with a history of hypertension and hyperlipidemia who presents with exertional left sided chest pain…"

Step 2: The Body of the HPI
Now that the topic sentence has been outlined it's time to delve into the structure of the body of the HPI. This may be less formulaic, as every patient and every story is different, but knowledge of the basic structural options is helpful for writing an eloquent HPI and doing it with some degree of speed.

Most commonly, when the story permits, HPIs are written in a chronological order beginning with the oldest directly relevant information and working towards the present time (in clinic).

According to this style, after the topic sentence, the HPI will mention any directly related medical history. This summary sentence or two at the beginning brings the reader up-to-date on the patient's current medical status. For example, if a patient is presenting with shortness of breath, it would be extremely helpful and informative (for the reader) if you briefly summarized any recent hospital admissions. The first two sentences may appear like this:

"Jane Doe is a 61 year old female with a history of smoking (40 pack years) who presents with shortness of breath. She was admitted 1 week ago for an acute exacerbation of COPD and discharged on tapered prednisone and azithromycin…"

Providing this summary of any recent and directly related healthcare encounters updates the reader on the patient's current medical status. Writing this summary is an acquired skill and one that you will learn in time as you write more HPIs and understand more about clinical medicine.

This summary sentence is especially important for follow-up visits. For example, in a patient presenting for high blood pressure follow-up, the first two sentences may appear like this:

"John Doherty is a 48 y.o. male who presents for hypertension follow-up. At his last visit 3 weeks ago we increased his dose of metoprolol from 50 mg BID to 100 mg BID…"

This second sentence summarizes the last clinic visit and updates the reader on the patient's current state prior to arrival in clinic today. The sentences to follow will then describe how he has been feeling since that last clinic visit in a chronological fashion.

The benefit of writing in this chronological style is that the HPI flows as a story, which makes it more memorable—there is a reason that much of history was recorded via oral accounts! It also makes it easy to think of sentence starters, as the day or date of significant events can be listed first. For example, in our example patient with chest pain, the first couple sentences in the HPI may look like this:

"John Doe is a 52 y.o. male with a history of hypertension and hyperlipidemia who presents with exertional left sided chest pain. 2 days ago he developed left sided chest pain rated as 3/10 while walking his dog. He has experienced similar pain since then, always while walking his dog and lasts until he returns home, sits down and takes a SL nitroglycerin. Today he was watching TV when experienced this same pain, though more severe and rated 8/10 and his wife called EMS for transport."

Note that the majority of text is spent describing the timeline for the patient's symptoms and how these symptoms changed over time. To write this, two of the three sentences simply started with the timeframe at which symptoms arose. Helpful key words when writing this section of the HPI include:

- Developed (e.g. 2 days ago he developed…)
- Experienced (e.g. this morning he experienced…)
- Noticed (e.g. he first noticed this pain 2 days ago while…)
- Began (e.g. symptoms began 2 days ago as…)

Typically, at least with chief complaints involving pain, there is some point in time at which symptoms become more severe and only then does the patient realize that they need to see a doctor. Here is another example for a patient with back pain:

"Adam Smith is a 43 year old male with a history of chronic back pain (on Norco) who presents with acute left low back pain. He was reportedly doing well and in his baseline health, taking 1 x Norco TID, until last night when he "tweaked" his back while lifting firewood. Since then the pain has been more acute, rated 9/10 and is constant. He wasn't able to sleep last night and presents for further evaluation and pain management."

Note the presence of relevant history in the first sentence, followed by a simple description of his pain. Then the second sentence gives us a picture of his usual state of health including how much Norco (a narcotic pain medication) he takes on a typical day. Now we are up-to-date on his usual state of health prior to last night. Then the following two sentences describe exactly why he is presenting to clinic—further evaluation and pain management given his severe 9/10 pain and consequent inability to sleep.

We often recommend that your HPI conveys, either implicitly or explicitly, exactly why the patient is presenting for evaluation. Implicit reasons for seeking medical attention are self-explanatory; that is, like acute pain, you easily understand why the patient is seeking help. Again, this often centers around some point in time at which pain becomes unbearable or more concerning.

Explicit reasons for seeking medical attention require that you state exactly why a patient is presenting for evaluation. For example, a patient might present following unprotected sexual intercourse to request STD testing even if they do not display symptoms. This desire for STD testing would need to be explicitly mentioned in the HPI because otherwise the reason for their ER visit would be unclear. So ultimately, your HPI should try and convey why the patient is seeking medical evaluation at that particular point in time.

And lastly, in our patient presenting for hypertension follow-up, the next couple sentences of the HPI may appear like this:

> "John Doherty is a 48 y.o. male who presents for hypertension follow-up. At his last visit 3 weeks ago we increased his dose of metoprolol from 50 mg BID to 100 mg BID. He has been feeling generally fatigued since then. On a couple occasions, typically in the morning, he has become light-headed and near-syncopal while standing up…"

The Body of the HPI: Deviations from the Pattern

Not all patients will have a nice, neat history that conforms to the HPI structure we have just described. Very simple complaints, very complex patients with more history needed than can be mentioned in a single line, and certain conditions in general may not conform. Some of this will be discovered on your own while working, but a few examples are listed below:

> "John Doe is a 12 m.o. male who presents with right ear tugging since last night."

This patient may not have a history of ear infections (otitis media). So this is not only a very simple complaint, but the patient has no prior history that may inform us as we read the rest of the HPI.

> "Jane Doe is a 78 y.o. female with a history of diabetes mellitus type II who presents with 5 hours of altered mental status."

Note this is missing the context at which symptoms arose, as not all conditions will have a single word to describe the setting of onset, and therefore this will be detailed in later sentences. In this case, it may be something along the lines of this:

"The pt was found dazed and disoriented by nursing facility staff before breakfast this morning…"

As is the nature of altered mental status (AMS) complaints, the patient is often unable to give a thorough and reliable history.

Step 3: The OPQRST Mnemonic
Once your HPI describes why the patient is presenting for evaluation (e.g. acute back pain), the next part of the HPI often includes greater description of their pain as summarized by the OPQRST mnemonic. This mnemonic stands for onset, palliation/provocation, quality, region/radiation, severity and timing. Each of these details describes something about the patient's pain as explained below:

Onset—onset describes the setting and time in which symptoms began. How long ago did symptoms begin? Did symptoms begin suddenly or gradually? What was the patient doing when symptoms began? Were they walking or running? Were they lying down or standing up? Did it occur after eating? Having all of these details is uncommon, but most patients provide some sort of description about when symptoms began and/or what they were doing at onset.

Palliative and Provocative factors—palliative refers to what makes the pain better and provocative means what makes the pain worse. For example, in a patient with leg pain, is it worse while bearing weight? Or is it worse simply with movement of the leg? In a patient with chest pain, is the pain worse while walking up stairs? Is it better while resting and lying down? Or is worse with deep breaths?

Quality—quality is the description of the pain. What does it feel like? Does it feel sharp or dull? Achy or burning? Crampy? Pressure-like? Stabbing? These words all describe different types of pain.

Region/Radiation—R can be used to mean either region or radiation (though radiation is more common because it is expected that you describe the region of a patient's pain). Region describes the primary location of pain and radiation describes the secondary region that pain sometimes extends towards or in to. In a patient with chest pain, is it located in the left chest, right chest, or substernal region? Does it radiate to the back, arm or neck? In a patient with low back pain, is it left sided or right sided? And does it radiate from the low back down one of the legs?

Severity—severity is either a word or a numerical score for the quantity of pain. When using words as descriptors, the spectrum includes slight, mild, moderate, severe, and excruciating. Sometimes a pain scale from 1-10 is used. 1/10 pain is near nothing; 10/10 pain is the most severe pain imaginable. You can also use patient quotes to describe this if the patient doesn't give you a nice clean answer (e.g. "horrible" pain).

Timing—timing refers to the frequency of symptoms. Is pain constant or does it come-and-go? Come-and-go is more technically known as intermittent. Review the table earlier in this chapter that provides terms for describing the frequency of symptoms; this provides a good list of concise descriptors including constant, waxing and waning, intermittent and episodic.

Some people add an "A" onto the end of the OPQRST mnemonic for Associated symptoms (i.e. **OPQRSTA)**. Associated symptoms refers to additional symptoms that the patient may have in addition to pain. Common associated symptoms include a fever, chills, nausea, vomiting, diarrhea, etc.

You certainly don't have to write the HPI in "OPQRST" order; in fact, it makes more sense to use a different order. OPQRST is simply a method to double-check that you included all of the important information in your HPI. The location of a patient's pain is often described first, as we recommend you do in the first sentence. Then the body of the HPI follows the timeline for a patient's symptoms and may include a few of the OPQRST descriptions. Once you have told the patient's "story," then you can use the OPQRSTA mnemonic to fill-in additional details. It may seem difficult to include all of these details in a single well-written paragraph, but you can often condense many of these descriptors into a single sentence or two. For example: "…pain is sharp, located over the epigastrium, and worse after eating." The HPIs for our patients with chest pain and back pain, according to this method, would look like this:

"John Doe is a 52 y.o. male with a history of hypertension and hyperlipidemia who presents with exertional left sided chest pain. 2 days ago (**O**nset) he developed left sided chest pain rated as 3/10 (**S**everity) while walking his dog. He has experienced similar pain since then, always while walking his dog (**O**) and lasts until he returns home, sits down and takes a SL nitroglycerin (**P**alliative). Today he was watching TV when experienced this same pain (**O**), though more severe and rated 8/10 (**S**) and his wife called EMS for transport. He was given 2 x nitroglycerin in route with improvement in pain from 7/10 to 3/10 (**P**). Upon arrival his pain is localized to the left chest (**R**egion and **R**adiation), rated 3/10 (**S**), dull in quality (**Q**uality). There has not been any associated diaphoresis or dyspnea with these bouts. No peripheral edema, weight gain, jaw or arm pain. No fevers, cough or other complaints (**A**ssociated symptoms)…"

"Adam Smith is a 43 year old male with a history of chronic back pain (on Norco) who presents with acute left low back pain. He was reportedly doing well and in his baseline health, taking 1 x Norco TID, until last night (**O**) when he "tweaked" his back while lifting firewood. Since then the pain has been more acute, rated 9/10 (**S**) and is constant (**T**). He wasn't able to sleep last night (**A**) and presents for further evaluation and pain management. Pain is described as sharp (**Q**) and does not radiate (**R**). It is worse with any bending movements and better while lying down (**P/P**). He denies any bowel or bladder incontinence. No saddle anesthesia (**A**)…"

Note that in both HPIs a couple OPQRST items were described during the chronological section, but once the patient presumably arrives to clinic, then we fill out the remainder of the OPQRST items—and we do so in 1-2 sentences. You can start this sentence, as we did in the first HPI, by writing: "On arrival, his pain is…" This thereby denotes that all further descriptions represent his current pain (at the time the physician is evaluates him). Once we fully described the patient's pain and check off all known OPQRST components, then we move on to describe associated symptoms.

There are other common details that don't fall into the OPQRSTA mnemonic. Assuming you are listening closely to the provider's questions, these should be easy to catch as they are quite obvious. Some common examples include:

1. **Has the patient had this type of pain before?** This is a common question for patients with a chief complaint involving pain (chest pain, abdominal pain, etc.). Pain that is completely new for a patient is typically more concerning than pain that a patient has had several times previously.

2. **What other concerns does the patient have?** Are they concerned about a particular disease process? Sometimes a patient will present for evaluation not because their symptoms are severe, but because they are concerned that their symptoms might represent a severe illness, so you may want to explicitly mention the patient's concerns in the HPI (e.g. appendicitis in a patient with abdominal pain).

3. **What treatment was attempted prior to arrival?** Did they take any medications at home? For example, in a patient with substernal chest pain, did they take Tums? And did this help or have no effect? If Tums alleviated the patient's pain in this case, then this would suggest that the cause is heartburn, not something more

serious.

Sometimes chief complaints will not involve pain (like our hypertension follow-up). Therefore not all of the components of OPQRSTA will be applicable, but it still serves as a good method to double check against your HPI. If pain is not the chief complaint, try and follow the doctor's questioning to guide the flow of your writing.

Step 4: Writing the End of the HPI

Once you have found your way to the present time in the patient's history and fully described the chief complaint (with the remaining OPQRSTA details), then the remainder of the HPI becomes somewhat chaotic. We will mention a couple ways to give this section some organization and keep it from being completely disorganized.

First, it is often preferable to mention any positives before you mention any negatives. This means, list symptoms that the patient DOES have before listing symptoms that the patient DOES NOT have. We call these pertinent positives and pertinent negatives, respectively. Physicians don't passively listen to patients as they provide the history for their chief complaint, but they listen and ask particular questions. Often times a physician will ask whether a patient has certain associated symptoms, depending on the chief complaint. If the patient admits to having one of these symptoms, then mention this symptom in your HPI before you list the symptoms that the patient denied having. This is most important when the list of pertinent negatives is especially long

You can see from the HPIs on the previous pages that that there were several symptoms that the patient did NOT have listed at the very end. These are called pertinent negatives. Typically, they are questions that the physician asks the patient to help narrow down their differential diagnosis (i.e. the mental list of possible causes for the patient's symptoms). Our recommendation is that you group this potentially long list of pertinent negatives by the condition the physician may be concerned about. This is often intuitive if you follow the order that the physician asked the question, as they will typically try and follow a single train of thought. For example, let's look at the two previous HPIs:

(Chest pain) "…There has not been any associated diaphoresis or dyspnea with these bouts. No peripheral edema, weight gain, jaw or arm pain. No fevers, cough or other complaints."

(Back pain) "He denies any bowel or bladder incontinence. No saddle anesthesia (**A**)…"

Notice how diaphoresis (excessive sweating) and dyspnea (difficulty breathing) were listed together. Patients may experience these two symptoms along with chest pain during a heart attack (a.k.a. an acute myocardial infarction). Weight gain, specifically due to peripheral edema (also mentioned), is due to heart failure, an insufficiency of the heart to pump blood. Neck and arm pain may occur in some patients having a heart attack, so they too would be concerning for a heart condition. So again, "No peripheral edema, weight gain, jaw or arm pain" are listed together because they are related to a potential cardiac etiology. Lastly, the patient denied having "fevers, cough or other complaints." The lungs and conditions like pneumonia and pulmonary embolism can also cause chest pain, so these pertinent negatives suggest that both of these lung conditions are less likely.

The back pain HPI is more straightforward because all of the symptoms mentioned pertain to a concerning albeit rare condition called cauda equina syndrome.

It may be difficult to make the connection between particular symptoms and the condition they may be suggestive of when you are first starting out, but hopefully later chapters will help you make some of these connections and write a more fluid HPI. However, you can almost always group symptoms together based on the timing and grouping in which the physician asked each question.

Following the list of pertinent positives and negatives at the end of the HPI, the very end of the HPI—either in the same paragraph or in a completely new paragraph—can be used to describe some supplemental information. This may describe further information about the patient's past medical history than is possible in the first (topic) sentence. For example, the very end of our sample HPIs looked like this:

> (Chest pain) "… No fevers, cough or other complaints. No history of diabetes or smoking. No family history of early cardiac events. No history of similar symptoms."

> (Back pain) "… No saddle anesthesia. He has previously received cortisone injections without relief. His last physical therapy visit was 1 year ago following an admission for acute back pain."

These last parcels of information often reiterate important aspects of the patient's past medical, social and family history. Because of the topic sentence, we already knew that the chest pain patient had two risk factors for heart disease (hypertension and hyperlipidemia), but what about the remaining three risk factors? The end of the HPI therefore addresses these additional risk factors (diabetes, history of smoking, family history of heart disease), which copies information technically found in the past medical history, social history, and family history.

In the back pain patient, the end of the HPI provided some additional information about his chronic back pain and what therapies (cortisone injections and physical therapy) that he has attempted in the past.

So any pertinent past medical, surgical, social or family history can be elaborated upon at the very end of the HPI to provide a more thorough history for the patient—this saves future readers from missing important pieces of the patient's history or at least saves them time as they read your note.

And with that, we have officially completed the HPIs for both the chest pain and back pain patients. This is how the HPIs for each patient now appear, in full:

Chest pain:

> "John Doe is a 52 y.o. male with a history of hypertension and

hyperlipidemia who presents with exertional left sided chest pain. 2 days ago he developed left sided chest pain rated as 3/10 while walking his dog. He has experienced similar pain since then, always while walking his dog and lasts until he returns home, sits down and takes a SL nitroglycerin. Today he was watching TV when experienced this same pain, though more severe and rated 8/10 and his wife called EMS for transport. He was given 2 x nitroglycerin in route with improvement in pain from 7/10 to 3/10. Upon arrival his pain is localized to the left chest, rated 3/10, dull in quality. There has not been any associated diaphoresis or dyspnea with these bouts. No peripheral edema, weight gain, jaw or arm pain. No fevers, cough or other complaints. No history of diabetes or smoking. No family history of early cardiac events. No history of similar symptoms."

Back pain:

"Adam Smith is a 43 year old male with a history of chronic back pain (on Norco) who presents with acute left low back pain. He was reportedly doing well and in his baseline health, taking Norco TID, until last night when he "tweaked" his back while lifting firewood. Since then the pain has been more acute, rated 9/10 and is constant. He wasn't able to sleep last night and presents for further evaluation and pain management. Pain is described as sharp and does not radiate. It is worse with any bending movements and better while lying down. He denies any bowel or bladder incontinence. No saddle anesthesia. He has previously received cortisone injections without relief. His last physical therapy visit was 1 year ago following an admission for acute back pain."

And for our patient presenting for hypertension follow-up, according to the same methodology, the full HPI may look like this:

"John Doherty is a 48 y.o. male who presents for hypertension follow-up. At his last visit 3 weeks ago we increased his dose of metoprolol from 50 mg BID to 100 mg BID. He has been feeling generally fatigued since then. On several occasions he has become light-headed and near-syncopal while standing up. These occur near-daily, typically in the morning. He denies any vertiginous symptoms. No nausea or vomiting. No palpitations. No history of similarly frequent symptoms. He denies any significant dietary changes since his last visit."

Step 5: Writing with Style in the HPI

Now that the basic structure and flow of the HPI has been described as above, we want to provide a brief introduction regarding the proper style of writing in the HPI. Medical notes are not written with superfluous words, but neither should they be so devoid of transitional words that it lacks readability and flow. It is the balance between these two extremes that we strive for in medical notes.

You have already been exposed to the general style of medical writing in the HPI throughout this chapter, but we can more explicitly describe some of this sentence structure.

Changing a Patient's Words into Medical Terminology

One of the easiest ways to reduce the number of words required in a note is to use medical terms for a patient's complaint. Patients typically describe their symptoms with no medical background to inform their word choice. You, on the other hand, will have an extra selection of words to help condense these complaints. For example, a female patient that presents with a burning sensation while she urinates as well as the sensation of having to urinate often, which actually causes her to urinate more than usual, may be described as having urinary urgency, frequency and dysuria. Those few words effectively summarize her symptoms and save a considerable amount of space in your HPI. Much of this summarization is tied to the process of learning medical terminology and your ability to efficiently describe symptoms in this manner will improve in time. Some of the most useful translational terms are listed on the following page:

Diaphoresis	Excessive sweating (often while at rest); this may be a sign of a heart attack
Dyspnea	Difficulty breathing

Dysuria	Pain—typically described as a burning sensation—during urination
Emesis	Vomit (noun)
Hematemesis	Bloody vomit
Hematochezia	Bright red blood passed rectally
Hematuria	Blood in the urine
Melena	Dark, tarry or coffee-ground appearing stool; it is a sign of upper GI (i.e. stomach, small intestine) bleeding.
Near-syncope	The sensation that one might lose consciousness
Palpitations	A subjective sense that a person's heartbeat is irregular
Paresthesias	Numbness or tingling sensation
Phonophobia	Sensitivity to sound
Photophobia	Sensitivity to light
Sputum	Mucus that has been coughed up
Syncope	Loss of consciousness; to "pass out" or "black out"
Urinary frequency	Frequent urination
Urinary urgency	The sensation of having to urinate often

Note that translating a patient's words into medical terms should not be done in legal, criminal or psychiatric cases, as described under the "Liability" section to follow.

Patient Pronouns

Sentences may often begin with the words "patient" or "he/she." The HPI is all about the patient, so it makes sense that we use these words frequently. For example, sentences may begin like this: "He was last here for a physical exam..." and "His hospital work-up showed..." In general, using a mixture of pronouns produces better flow and readability than starting every sentence with the same identifier ("pt reports that... pt thinks...pt complains...")—this will get really stale, really fast. Excessive use of the word "patient" will be particularly noticeable because of the hard consonant ("P"); in addition, HPIs that use the word "patient" excessively may seem impersonal. For those reasons, we recommend limiting your use of the word "patient" and instead using "he", "she", "his", or "her" in your HPI.

Fragments are your friend

On a similar note to the point above, sentences may also begin with the symptom you're describing—this can help you avoid overuse of the word "patient." For example, if a patient is complaining of chest pain you may write, "Pain is located over the left chest without radiation to the left arm, neck or back." This uses fewer words than starting the sentence with the words "the patient describes the pain as…"

If a patient is denying a long list of symptoms, just starting the sentence with the word "no" is also helpful. This is particularly helpful for pertinent negatives that are tacked onto the end of the HPI. Again, an example for a patient with chest pain patient denying multiple symptoms may look like this:

> "Denies shortness of breath or peripheral edema. No fevers, cough, cold or other infectious symptoms. No history of hyperlipidemia, hypertension, diabetes or smoking."

As should be evident, the advantage of using fragments is that unnecessary words are eliminated, producing a more concise HPI with only the words vital to our understanding still remaining. This is not a style that an English professor would approve of, but medical notes are not written by English professors, and despite the habit to write in grammatically correct sentences, fragments can be quite helpful to have in the medical scribe's toolbox—primarily at the end of the HPI.

Another Sentence Starter: Time

The last formulaic type of sentence starter is simply the time at which a symptom began. It is not only easy to follow, but easy to write an HPI by merely following the time frame of the story and starting sentences with the time of onset. For example, if a patient presents with abdominal pain according to a classical though condensed appendicitis progression, the format could be:

> "*3 days ago* the pt first noticed a diffuse periumbilical abdominal pain. *The following day,* she became nauseated and vomited on several occasions. *Since waking at 0400* this morning she has experienced fever, chills, loss of appetite and sharp abdominal pain localized to the RLQ."

Liability and Psychiatric Complaints

There are some instances in which substituting medical terms for a patient's word choice and using fragmented sentences or other shortened writing forms are inappropriate. The primary instance of this is for chief complaints that may result in legal or criminal action (either against another person or against the treating physician). Common instances include physical assault, motor vehicle accidents, and psychiatric complaints. In these cases, using direct quotations is important. For example, in a physical assault case that may go to court (and which may use the medical note as evidence), a segment from the HPI may appear as follows:

> The patient reports that her husband returned home from work angry and "fuming" and called her a "bitch." She reports that she then asked him what was wrong and "he hit my head against the kitchen wall."

Quoting specific words used by the patient is very safe from a liability standpoint and is the gold standard in these cases. So if in doubt, use direct quotes!

You may have noticed that we did not include any psychiatric terms in the list of translational terms on the previous pages. This is because psychiatric complaints are often very unique. Therefore, the HPI for patients with psychiatric complaints like anxiety, depression or suicidal ideation will rely on quotations (not terms) to accurately portray the mental state of the patient.

Sample Doctor-Patient Interaction

Now that you have read about the methodology for writing an eloquent HPI, we have included a sample patient-doctor encounter here. Although following along with this transcript is easier than listening to the encounter, take notes as you read and then try your hand at writing an HPI for this patient in the space provided.

Doctor: What brings you in today?

Patient: Well, I've had some low back problems for the past few years and it really seems to be acting up today.

Doctor: Have you been doing anything like lifting weights, yard work, etc. that you think might have made it worse?

Patient: I have been moving a lot of boxes the last few days because I'm moving places right now.

Doctor: Did the pain begin suddenly while lifting a box or when did you first notice it?

Patient: I guess I did have a twinge while lifting a box yesterday, but it wasn't really that bad until I woke up this morning.

Doctor: Did you hear a pop or anything like that?

Patient: No

Doctor: Any recent falls?

Patient: Nope

Doctor: Ok. So where does it hurt. On the left? Right? Down low or up high? Can you show me?

Patient: It hurts in this area (gestures towards the right lumbar region)

Doctor: And how would you describe the pain? Sharp? Dull? Achy?

Patient: Probably sharp

Doctor: Does it hurt more when you bend over or move?

Patient: Yeah, definitely.

Doctor: And does the pain radiate down your legs?

Patient: Yeah, it goes down into my right leg to about here (patient gestures to pain running along the lateral right hip and stopping at the knee)

Doctor: So it stops at the knee? Correct? It doesn't go into the feet?

Patient: Yeah, I don't think it goes to the foot.

Doctor: Is it similar to back pain you've had before?

Patient: Yes, it's exactly the same, only worse.

Doctor: Did you have the pain into your leg before?

Patient: Yes

Doctor: What have you taken for the pain?

Patient: I took 3 ibuprofen this morning and that helped a little bit.

Doctor: Have you had any bowel or bladder problems?

Patient: What? No.

Doctor: Have you had any numbness when you wipe yourself or weakness in your legs?

Patient: Um… no.

Try writing your HPI for this patient here:

"Jonathon Doe is a 40 year old male _____

_____

_____

_____

_____

_____

_____

_____

_____

Here is the HPI that we wrote for this encounter:

"Jonathon Doe is a 40 year old male with a history low back pain who presents with progressive right low back pain. This began yesterday while lifting boxes at home. He had a sudden twinge of sharp pain at onset but pain was mild until he woke up this morning in more severe pain. He took 3 ibuprofen with only mild relief before presenting for pain management. Pain radiates down the lateral right thigh down to the knee but not into the foot. It is sharp, worse bending over, and similar to prior episodes of his back pain. No bowel or bladder problems. No numbness with wiping.

You should notice that we covered all of the OPQRST components in this paragraph. In addition, there are several somewhat unusual symptoms that the patient denied having. You will learn more about these "rule out" questions later, but essentially, back pain that causes bladder or bowel problems represents a more severe type of back pain called cauda equina syndrome, which the physician is making sure the patient does NOT have.

Additional complete HPIs are shown in the context of complete notes later in this book in Appendix A. For now, we will move on to documentation of the review of systems (ROS).

Review of Systems (ROS)

The Review of Systems is part of the subjective section of the medical note. In the primary care clinic, it may be obtained in one of two ways: the first is a form given to the patient after they register at the front desk in which they are told to check any symptoms that they are currently experiencing; the second is during the physician's conversation with the patient. When obtained by the doctor himself, it may be obtained during or shortly after the information for the history of present illness. It is minimally important compared to the HPI, but important details from this question list are often included at the end of the HPI (called pertinent positives or negatives).

The ROS is basically a list of questions that the doctor goes through with the patient. The main reason the ROS is performed is to complete billing requirements. Many patient visits require the documentation of at least 4 different bodily systems within the ROS to meet appropriate billing criteria; you can learn more about the exact requirements in the tables found in Chapter 12: Billing and Coding.

There are technically 14 body systems that make up the review of systems. These include the gastrointestinal system, respiratory system, cardiovascular system, etc. It is called the "review" of systems because the physician will ask questions about symptoms (e.g. nausea) within multiple body systems (e.g. the gastrointestinal system).

Some doctors will have a long, formal review of systems; some will have a core list of systems that they inquire about and they do this very quickly. Many scribes struggle with differentiating the review of systems from the physical exam. It may help you to think of the ROS as the review of *symptoms* rather than the review of *systems*. This means that the ROS includes only symptoms verbally mentioned by the patient; remember, it is included in the "Subjective" section of the medical note and therefore is based on information provided by the patient. The physical exam, in contrast, is part of the "Objective" section and includes *findings* (not *symptoms*) on part of the physician during the exam of the patient.

In primary care, the review of systems may be completed via a checklist given to the patients, in which they will check any symptoms that they are currently experiencing, or the physician may ask questions that are related to the review of systems. These questions may be phrased like this:

"Have you had any changes in your weight recently?"

If the patient says that he has gained weight recently (for whatever reason), then you would document this as follows:

Review of Systems
Constitutional: + weight gain

Or

Review of Systems
Constitutional: POSITIVE weight gain

If the patient denies any recent changes in weight, then you will see it documented using either the word "denies _____" or "no _____" as shown below:

Review of Systems
Constitutional: No changes in weight

Your goal is to be able to appropriately affix a symptom like weight gain to the corresponding bodily system (the constitutional system in this case).

The full list of systems and the symptoms within each system are listed on the following pages. We have tried to define the most common terms that you may encounter and left other more obscure terms out. Many of these terms will overlap with the translational terms used in the HPI, although the ROS tends to be even more technical and therefore there are more terms listed here than in the prior section. Terms that are largely self-explanatory are labeled with the abbreviation SE.

1. General/Constitutional System

The constitutional system refers to symptoms that are non-specific to one of the bodily systems. Many of these symptoms occur in a variety of illnesses. For example, any infection (of the lungs, skin, mouth, etc.) may result in a fever and therefore a "fever" is considered a general symptom.

Changes in weight	Weight gain or loss
Chills	Sense of feeling cold and shivering for no apparent reason. Sometimes called "shaking chills"
Fatigue	Feeling unusually tired
Fever	Temperature above 100.4 F
Malaise	Feeling generally unwell
Myalgias	Body aches ("myo" referring to muscle and "algia" referring to pain)

2. Head

Headache	SE
Light-headedness	A type of dizziness

3. Eyes

Redness	SE
Watery eyes	SE
Discharge	Fluid drainage from the eye
Diplopia	Double vision ("Di" referring to two and "–plopia" referring to vision)
Blurry vision	Fuzzy vision
Photophobia	Sensitivity of the eyes to light; often occurs with migraine headaches

4a. Ears (Combined in the ENT system)

Hearing loss	SE
Otalgia	Ear pain ("oto" refers to the ears and "algia" refers to pain)
Otorrhea	Ear discharge ("oto" refers to the ears and "-rrhea"

| | means discharge) |
| Tinnitus | Ringing in an ear or ears. Pronounced "tin-ih-tis" |

4b. Nose (Combined in the ENT system)

Congestion	Nasal stuffiness
Epistaxis	Bloody nose
Rhinorrhea	Runny nose ("rhino" refers to the nose and "-rrhea" means discharge)
Sneezing	SE

4c. Throat (Combined in the ENT system)

Dental pain	SE
Dysphagia	Difficulty swallowing ("dys" meaning abnormal and "phagia" referring to the act of swallowing)
Hoarseness	A raspy or strained voice
Snoring	Loud, snorting or grunting sounds made while sleeping
Sore throat	SE

5. Cardiovascular

Chest pain	SE
Diaphoresis	Excessive sweatiness, typically in the setting of chest pain due to a heart attack
Lower extremity edema	Swelling (edema) typically occurring in the ankles because of heart failure or poor venous blood flow
Orthopnea	Shortness of breath while lying down ("ortho" means straight and "-pnea" refers to breathing)
Palpitations	A subjective sense that a person's heartbeat is irregular; it may be described as fast, pounding, slow, irregular, etc.

6. Respiratory

Cough	SE
Dyspnea	Nearly synonymous with difficulty breathing ("dys" means abnormal and "-pnea' refers to breathing)
Shortness of breath	SE
Sputum	A productive cough is one in which a patient expels sputum while coughing. Sputum color (clear, brown, yellow or green) can be informative in diagnosing the underlying cause
Wheezing	A high pitched whistling sound heard while breathing, typically while exhaling

7. Gastrointestinal

Abdominal pain	SE
Constipation	Infrequent bowel movements (BMs)
Diarrhea	Loose or watery bowel movements (BMs)
Dysphagia	Difficulty swallowing
Hematochezia	Bright red blood passed rectally
Melena	Dark, tarry or coffee-ground stools
Nausea	The sensation that one might vomit
Vomiting	SE

8a. Genitourinary

Dysuria	Painful urination, often described as burning
Erectile dysfunction	Inability to develop or maintain an erection
Hematuria	Blood in the urine
Nocturia	The necessity to urinate overnight; often seen in aging males
Oliguria	Decreased urine output
Polyuria	Increased urine output
Urinary frequency	The act of urinating frequently
Urinary incontinence	Loss of bladder control

Urinary urgency	Sensation that one has to urinate frequently or immediately when the sensation arises

8b. Genitourinary (female):

Irregular menses	Abnormal number of days between menstrual periods
Itching	SE
Menopause	The phase during which a female's menses become irregular and eventually cease altogether
Vaginal bleeding	SE
Vaginal discharge	SE

9. Musculoskeletal

Joint pain	SE
Spasm	A sudden, involuntary muscle contraction
Stiffness	Rigidity; moving with difficulty
Swelling	SE

10. Skin

Dryness	Dry skin
Lacerations	Cuts in the skin
Lesions	Openings in the skin; sores
Pruritus	Itching or itchiness
Rashes	Redness of the skin

11. Neurological

Memory changes	SE
Paralysis	Complete loss of motor function
Paresis	Reduced muscle function
Paresthesias	Numbness/tingling sensation
Seizures	Abnormal brain activity often resulting in convulsive movements and/or changes in mental processes

Syncope	Loss of consciousness
Vertigo	Dizziness described as a spinning sensation; different than light-headedness
Weakness	Lacking usual strength

12. Psychiatric

Anxiety	Excessive uneasiness or worry that is out of proportion to a circumstance
Depression	Prolonged sadness and/or dejection
Homicidal ideation	Thoughts of killing others
Suicidal ideation	Thoughts of killing oneself

The 12 systems listed above represent the core systems used in most review of systems templates. There are a few other more obscure systems that may be used by specialists as shown here:

13. Hematologic

This refers to disorders of the blood and the most common symptom for the hematologic system is easy bleeding and/or easy bruising. Some medications may "thin" a patient's blood and cause easy bleeding or bruising.

14. Endocrine

The endocrine system refers to symptoms that suggest an underlying hormonal imbalance. Major structures of the endocrine system include the hypothalamus, pituitary, and adrenal glands. Common symptoms in the endocrine symptom include:

Intolerance to heat or cold	Suggestive of thyroid dysfunction
Polyuria	Excessive urination
Polydipsia	Excessive thirst
Polyphagia	Excessive hunger

The three P's above are a sign of high blood sugar in a patient with diabetes mellitus, which is related to an insufficiency of the hormone insulin.

Medications

After the review of systems the doctor will often review the patient's medication list. This review is sometimes performed by nursing staff and updated in the patient's record before the physician sees the patient. The electronic medical record will likely require that any medication listed includes the these details:

1. **Medication name** – medications typically have a generic and brand name. Generic medication names are written in all lower case letters (e.g. warfarin) and brand names are written with the first letter capitalized (e.g. Coumadin).

2. **Route** – the method by which the medication is delivered to the body. Medications may be given orally (PO), intramuscularly (IM), intravenously (IV), or sublingually (beneath the tongue; SL). Nearly all medications taken at home are in the oral form and therefore this may not be specified in the medication list.

3. **Dose** – the amount of medication taken at any one time. Most oral medications are dosed in milligrams.

4. **Frequency** – the number of times per day that a patient takes a particular medication. You will see the abbreviations QD, BID, TID and QID instead of the words once daily, twice daily, three times daily, and four times daily. The combination of dose and frequency is called "**dosage**" (see below)

5. **Compliance** – if a patient has a prescribed medication on their medication list, it does not mean that they take the medication as prescribed. Patients that do not take medications as prescribed are called "non-compliant." For this reason, there may be place to describe whether the patient is compliant or non-compliant with their medication regimen.

Medications:

Medication	Dosage	Dispense	Refill
amoxicillin	500 mg TID	30	0
aspirin	81 mg QD	0	0
omeprazole (Prilosec)	20 mg QD	30	2
simvastatin (Zocor)	20 mg QD	30	2

Medication Allergies

Severe allergic reactions can result in a condition called anaphylaxis, which can be life-threatening if not immediately treated. Therefore, the electronic medical record will have a section dedicated to listing a patient's medication allergies and possibly other allergies as well (foods, pollens, pets, etc.). Any medication or item in a patient's allergy list should include the type of reaction induced by that item. The most severe reactions are anaphylaxis and angioedema (swelling of tissues beneath the skin; if it affects the lips, mouth or throat it may result in asphyxiation). However, there are many more mild forms of allergies including some reactions that may be described as an "intolerance" rather than a true "allergy." Examples of symptoms that may represent a medication intolerance include nausea, dizziness, or altered mental status after taking a particular medication.

Some of the most common medication allergies include:
1. Penicillins – penicillin was the first antibiotic discovered and mass produced. It belongs to a class of antibiotics called beta-lactam antibiotics and related medications include amoxicillin and ampicillin.
2. Sulfa – sulfa refers to a group of substances that contain a sulfonamide group. The antibiotic Bactrim (trimethoprim-sulfamethoxazole) is the one common antibiotic that patients with a sulfa allergy cannot take.

Past Medical History (PMHx)

The past medical history includes all problems that the patient has had in the past. For complex patients, this list may include dozens of different conditions. The term "Problem list" is a closely related term except that whereas the past medical history includes all prior conditions, the problem list only includes current or chronic conditions—those conditions that affect the patient at the present point in time.

Most electronic medical records allow you to choose the diagnosis that you wish to add to the past medical history and then it may allow you to insert the date of onset and any desired comments. Listing a brief comment in the past medical history next to a particular condition can be very helpful for future healthcare professionals when they review a patient's chart. An example of a patient's past medical history and problem list may appear like this:

Past Medical History:

Diagnosis	Date	Comments
Hypertension		
Breast lump	2011	
Hodgkin's disease, of lymph nodes of head, face, and neck	2011	Dx'd 2011 via biopsy, tx'd with chemo and radiation; in remission
Tobacco use disorder		
LVH (left ventricular hypertrophy)	4/9/2013	
CAD (coronary artery disease)	6/12/2013	80% stenosis of distal RCA, tx'd with drug-eluting stent
Distal radius fracture, left	2009	

Problem List:

Problem	Comments
Hypertension	On amlodipine, metoprolol
Tobacco use disorder	1 ppd smoker
LVH (left ventricular hypertrophy)	
CAD (coronary artery disease)	s/p distal RCA stenting; annual FU with cardiology

Past Surgical History (PSHx)

The past surgical history is sometimes regarded as a subheading of the past medical history or it may be a separate section of the note altogether. It is a simple accounting of all surgeries and procedures the patient has had in the past. Many of the technical names for a particular surgery will incorporate one of these three suffixes:

1. –ectomy: removal of (e.g. appendectomy)
2. –otomy: to cut into (e.g. tracheotomy)
3. –ostomy: to make an artificial opening, often an hole (e.g. colostomy)

Surgical History:

Procedure	Date
Hx coronary stent placement	6/13/2013
Open reduction internal fixation (ORIF), left radius	5/7/2009

Social History (SHx)

The social history consists of habits (smoking, alcohol, drug use) and social situation (living in nursing home? alone? feel safe at home?). This section is highly important in the primary care setting. Some of these details are not always medically important, but they help the physician to build a rapport with the patient. On the other hand, some details here may be pertinent to the patient's medical care. Knowing where they live, for example, may be important in an elderly person that comes in with 10 lbs of weight loss in the last 6 months, as that may suggest to the doctor (and future readers of your note) that the patient may not be caring for themselves adequately at home. You will encounter more specific examples of important social history details during your clinical training, but a list of potentially important social history details is given here:

- Living situation (home by self, nursing home, etc.)
- Number of children
- Number of siblings
- Hobbies and what they do for exercise
- Job position (e.g. mechanic at the nearby Toyota plant)
- Marital status (Married? Divorced? Single?)

- Recent life events
- Smoking status (never smoker, previous smoker, active smoker)
- Alcohol use (none, socially, 3 beers per day, etc.)

Family History (FHx)

The family history recorded by primary care providers is more comprehensive than any other healthcare setting. At the minimum it will include the medical history of direct family members (mother, father, brother, sister) but may also expand out to more indirect relatives (aunt, uncle, grandmother, grandfather). Family medicine and primary care are really the main purveyors of preventative medicine. The task of the general practitioner in these settings is to provide "risk factor modification." For example, hyperlipidemia ("high blood lipids") is a risk factor for stroke and a heart attack. To reduce the risk of these events, the primary care physician will likely suggest a medication to lower a patient's lipids and/or cholesterol levels and thereby reduce the likelihood of a heart attack or stroke.

Noting a patient's familial risk factors is important because it may lower the threshold that the physician has for modifying other risk factors. Using the same example of stroke as above, if a patient has a family history of stroke in his father (at a reasonably young age, like 60 years old), the doctor may be more inclined to treat the patient's borderline hyperlipidemia with a medication because, if left untreated, it would further increase his risk of a stroke. The most common conditions regarding family medical history are listed below. Some are risk factors for other diseases (like hypertension, hyperlipidemia, and diabetes are for heart attacks and strokes) whereas others are life-threatening in-and-of themselves (like heart attacks and strokes). Colon, breast and prostate cancer are especially significant in the primary clinic as they will affect the age at which a patient starts being monitored for these conditions via colonoscopy, mammography, and PSA testing, respectively.

- Diabetes mellitus
- Hypertension
- Hyperlipidemia
- Heart attack – this is most important for male family members before age 55 and female family members before age 65.

- Stroke
- Colon cancer
- Breast cancer (females only)
- Prostate cancer (males only)

Physical Exam

The next major task for the medical scribe is accurate documentation of the physical exam. The physical exam is the first part of the objective section of the medical note. It is "objective" in the sense that it describes the physician's unbiased and therefore objective findings. Remember, the review of systems is based on *symptoms* reported by the patient; the physical exam is based on *findings* as discovered by the physician.

Different EMRs have different ways in which you will document the physical exam, including either check boxes or free-text areas. Check boxes work well for documenting normal findings, but free-text is far superior (both in terms of speed and level of detail) for documenting abnormal findings.

Some physicians will choose to verbally report their findings as they perform the exam while others will summarize any abnormal findings with you after leaving the patient's room. This is normally a matter of preference, though sometimes it can seem insensitive to discuss certain findings within the patient's presence (like their hygiene, or maybe findings on a pelvic exam).

Your goal is to be able to observe the physician's examinations and then document the appropriate finding(s) in the patient's note. So for example, when the physician takes the otoscope to look into the patient's ear, what are they looking at? What does a normal examination of the ear include as findings? Individual physical exam sections in this chapter will detail normal physical exam findings and some common abnormal findings.

The normal physical exam is usually performed or at least documented in a head-to-toe manner. The exam may be comprehensive (including genital and rectal exams) for visits like annual physical exams or the exam may be focused on only a couple specific exam sections for acute care visits (e.g. a chief complaint of ankle pain).

The following page demonstrates the complete normal physical exam with acceptable abbreviations. It may seem overwhelming when seen in its entirety, but the majority of patient visits will not require documentation of full genitourinary (GU), pelvic, breast, rectal, and neurologic exams. On the pages to follow we have broken down the exam piece-by-piece with explanations of common terminology.

Full Physical Exam

BP 122/66 | Pulse 103 | Temp 95.7 °F (35.4 °C) | Resp 16 | Ht 1.626 m (5' 4") | Wt 66.225 kg (146 lb) | BMI 25.06 kg/m2 | SpO2 91% | LMP 03/21/2013 | Breastfeeding? No

GENERAL: Patient is pleasant, comfortable appearing, no acute distress.

ENT: Normocephalic, atraumatic. Oropharynx normal, no erythema. Tonsillar pillars wnl, no exudate. TMs clear bilaterally. External canals normal.

EYES: No conjunctival injection, no significant icterus, PERRL, EOMI.

NECK: Supple. No lymphadenopathy, thyromegaly, JVD or carotid bruit.

RESPIRATORY: Lungs are CTA without rales or rhonchi. Good air movement.

CARDIOVASCULAR: Regular rate and rhythm. No murmurs, rubs or gallops. Radial and dorsalis pedis pulses are 2+ and symmetric. Good capillary refill. No lower extremity edema.

GI: Soft, non-distended without hepatosplenomegaly. Non-tender without rebound or guarding. BS are normal.

GU (male): Normal external genitalia. No scrotal swelling or tenderness of the testes. No genital lesions.

PELVIC (female): Normal external genitalia. Physiologic vaginal discharge within the vaginal vault. No adnexal mass or tenderness. No cervical motion tenderness.

BREAST (female): No palpable masses. No dimpling or erythema of the skin. No nipple discharge. Normal axillary nodes.

RECTAL: No fistula or fissure. No external hemorrhoids. No mass on digital exam. Normal appearing, occult-negative stool. Guaiac negative stool. Normal, smooth, non-tender prostate (male only).

NEUROLOGIC: The patient is awake, alert and oriented x 3. 2+ biceps, brachioradialis, patellar and Achilles reflexes. Upper and lower extremity strength is 5/5 and symmetric.

PSYCHIATRIC: Good eye contact. Normal affect, normal speech.

SKIN: Exposed skin is within normal limits.

MS: No obvious muscular asymmetry. No CVA tenderness.

Generally speaking the physical exam can be divided into five different activities performed by the doctor:

1. Inspection – looking at a part of the body
2. Palpation – feeling or pushing on a body part
3. Auscultation – listening with a stethoscope
4. Percussion – tapping on part of the body and listening for changes in sound (related to the density of the object being percussed)
5. Special tests – this includes a large array of tests that don't fall into the above categories, especially those found in the neurological exam.

Vital Signs

The vital signs are the patient's blood pressure (BP), heart rate (HR), respiratory rate (RR), oximetry ("sats") and temperature. Not all patients will have all vital signs documented (like with really quick same-day appointments). Vital signs will usually be entered by the CMA or nurse and it is rare that the scribe will need to enter this into the medical record. That being said, it is nice to understand these numbers.

Blood Pressure (BP)

This is expressed as two numbers, stated as "x over y." For example a BP of 140/90 is stated as "140 over 90." These numbers represent the arterial blood pressure during systole (systolic blood pressure, SBP) and diastole, respectively. Normal blood pressure is age dependent. We use 120/80 as general guideline. High blood pressure is defined as a blood pressure higher than 140/90 on at least 3 separate clinic visits and this may be referred to as hypertension. For a truly accurate measure, patients must be resting comfortably for 5 minutes prior to testing and sit with the arm relaxed during testing, otherwise results may be skewed. In addition, repeat measurements are often taken and averaged together in the diagnosis of hypertension. Low blood pressure is dependent on several factors such as age; a blood pressure of less than 90/60 is considered low in an adult and may cause symptoms (light-headedness, syncope, etc.) if even lower. Low blood pressure is called hypotension.

Heart Rate (HR)

Defined as the number of beats per minute (bpm) of the heart. This also is age dependent and is generally higher for infants and children. For adults 90 bpm is borderline and above 100 bpm is generally accepted as fast; a fast heart rate is called tachycardia. In contrast, bradycardia is a slow heart rate. Technically the cut-off for bradycardia is less than 60 bpm, but this is actually normal in some people and asymptomatic in most; symptomatic bradycardia may occur at less than 50 bpm.

Respiratory Rate (RR)

Simply defined as the number of breaths per minute. Less than 12 is a slow respiratory rate and is called bradypnea (very rare); greater than 20 is a fast respiratory rate and called tachypnea (common).

Oximetry

Also known as pulse oximetry, this is a technique for measuring oxygenation of the blood. This utilizes the fact that oxygenated blood is red and deoxygenated blood is purple. Using a small probe attached to the patient's finger (or toe) and two different wavelengths of light, pulse oximetry estimates the percentage of oxygenated hemoglobin. 93-100% is considered normal; less than 90% is low and called hypoxia. You may hear it referred to as oxygen saturation or just "sats." Abbreviations for it include SpO2, SaO2 or sats.

Temperature

Body temperature be measured rectally, in the axillae (armpits), orally, or using ear or forehead probes. Usually the temperature is stated in both Fahrenheit and Celsius and the way in which the temperature was obtained is indicated. 98.6°F or 37°C is normal. A fever is defined as a temperature higher than 100.4°F (38°C).

General Appearance

Here the general appearance of the patient is documented, possibly just listed as "general." This part of the exam is documented in most patients and includes a description of comfort level, physical condition, and body position. Any general abnormalities may also be noted here, such as "walks with a cane." Common descriptors include:

- Thin or obese
- Comfortable or uncomfortable appearing
- Seated, standing or lying down
- No acute distress (NAD)

Head, Eyes, Ears, Nose and Throat (HEENT) Exam

This is a general outline of the exam findings for the listed body parts. This part of the exam is often only included in patients for whom the physician performs a comprehensive physical exam as part of an annual physical or patients who have a chief complaint that involves the head, eyes, ears, nose or throat.

Head (the "H" of HEENT)

- Normocephalic – normally shaped head
- Atraumatic – no head trauma (delete this in the case of a laceration, bruising, etc.)

Eyes ("E" of HEENT)

Essentially, this inspects the pupils for normal shape and function. Examples of a null (or completely normal) examination of the eyes may include:

- Pupils are equal, round, and reactive to light (abbreviated PERRL). This addresses the two variables below:
  - o Fixed vs reactive pupils – the pupils normally constrict (shrink) in response to light and this is called appropriate reactivity. Fixed pupils are those that do not react to light and are the sign of a serious intracranial abnormality.
  - o Constricted vs dilated pupils – the pupils are very small (constricted) or very large (dilated). The pupils may also be described by their size in millimeters to address this.
- Sclera are anicteric – there is no icterus (a.k.a. jaundice), or

yellowing, of the sclera (white of the eye), which occurs with liver failure.

- No conjunctival injection – injection refers to the presence of streaky redness in the eyes, typically indicative of conjunctivitis ("pink eye")
- Extra-ocular movements (or muscles) intact (EOMI) – the extra-ocular muscles are the muscles that control eye movement. The physician will have the patient follow their fingers as they move them in an "H" shape or other formation in front of the patient's eyes. If the patient performs this adequately, the exam finding is documented as "EOMI."

Ears ("E" of HEENT)

In the ears the most important exam item is the tympanic membrane (TM), the membrane that transmits sound to the middle. The most common abnormality of the TMs is otitis media (a.k.a. an ear infection), in which the normally clear TM will be red (due to inflammation).

Normal appearing TMs may be described as:
- Clear – the TMs are normally nearly translucent, but may become dull appearing or erythematous (red) in cases of effusions or infection, respectively
- TM is bulging – this may be due to fluid within the middle ear, pushing the TM outward
- Middle ear effusion – the accumulation of fluid behind a tympanic membrane

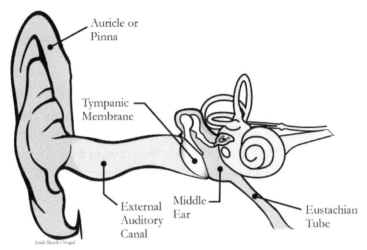

Figure 14: Anatomy of the ear

The auditory canals may also be mentioned if the physician is particularly concerned about "Swimmer's ear," known as otitis externa. This is an infection of the canal that connects the outer ear to the TM. Abnormal findings may include:

- External auditory canal is obstructed with cerumen (a.k.a. wax)
- External auditory canal is red and inflamed – otitis externa finding

Nose ("N" of HEENT)
Examination of the nose is typically only performed in patients complaining of sinus symptoms (rhinorrhea, congestion, tenderness). The exam will be performed using an otoscope and the exam is not overly helpful, but the physician may be able to see the nasal turbinates (bones covered with mucous membranes deep in the nose), which may be red and inflamed due to seasonal allergies or other inflammatory conditions. The nose may also be examined in children who may have placed something in a naris.

Throat ("T" of HEENT)
The oropharynx is the body part examined when the physician has the patient open his/her mouth and say "ah." It includes inspection of the oropharynx (back of the mouth) and tonsils. "Oropharynx within normal limits" is a common finding noted here. Erythema (redness), swelling and exudate (pus) are frequently noted. Also, the location of the uvula (usually

midline) may be noted; the uvula is the appendage that hangs down in the back of the throat.

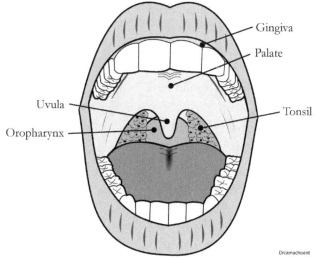

Figure 15: Anatomy of the oral cavity and oropharynx

Examples of oropharyngeal exam findings include:

- Moderate bilateral posterior oropharyngeal swelling with exudate, uvula is midline – there is some redness on both sides with some pus, but no large abscess that is pushing the uvula to one side.

- 2+ tonsils without evidence of exudate – the tonsils are enlarged but without any pus. The size of the tonsils is graded from 0 to 4+ with 0 meaning the tonsils fit within the tonsillar fossa, 4+ meaning the tonsils are dangerously large.

- White plaques on the tongue – due to a yeast infection of the mouth (thrush).

Dental exam

The dental exam is also included in the HEENT section of the physical exam. This includes the tooth numbering system, which is important for patients with dental complaints. A good way to remember this is to imagine the patient is facing you with his/her mouth open (as in the diagram below). The numbering system then starts in the patient's right rear (posterior) upper molars and progresses clockwise in the circle of teeth made by the open mouth.

The objects examined in the dental exam will include:

- Dentition – the overall arrangement and hygiene of the teeth. "Poor dentition" would be a common finding.
- Dental caries – cavities, which will often be tender to percussion when severe.
- Fluctuance – palpable fluid beneath the skin or mucous membranes. In the dental exam, the doctor will look for fluctuance as a sign of a dental abscess.

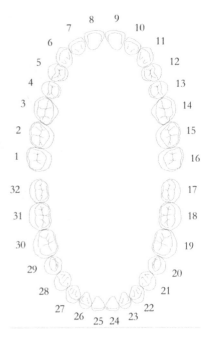

Figure 16: Dental numbering

Examination of the Neck

Usually involves visual inspection, palpation, and assessment of range of motion. Like most sections of the physical exam, it may not be performed in patients presenting for an unrelated complaint, though the neck is typically evaluated during an annual physical exam.

Common terms encountered in the neck exam include:

- Carotid bruit (pronounced "brew-e") – this is a sound heard upon auscultation of the carotid arteries in the neck. It is a turbulent sound that may be due to stenosis of these arteries.
- Jugular venous distention (JVD) – is an enlargement of the jugular veins on each side of the neck due to fluid overload, as occurs in right sided heart failure. No JVD is a common null finding.
- Lymphadenopathy (or just adenopathy) – refers to the enlargement of lymph nodes in the neck, commonly related to strep throat.
- Meningismus – a stiff, rigid neck with limited ROM in several directions, most commonly as a result of meningitis.
- Nuchal rigidity – neck stiffness, one characteristic of meningitis
- Supple – no restriction in range of motion.

100

- Tenderness – it is common to have tenderness over the muscles along the spine (paraspinous or paraspinal muscles) or potentially over the vertebral bodies as well (midline tenderness).
- Thyromegaly – enlargement of the thyroid, the gland that controls metabolic rate and is located beneath the Adam's apple; this may occur with hypothyroidism.

Respiratory exam

Refers to the examination of the lungs performed by the physician. This is an important part of the physical exam and is performed for most patients. The unremarkable exam may include these descriptors:

- Clear to auscultation – no abnormal sounds
- No rales, rhonchi, or wheezes – no evidence of one of the three most common pathological lung sounds
- Good air movement

Abnormalities may include:

- Significantly diminished air movement – poor air movement in and out of the lungs with each breath
- End-expiratory wheezes – the most common time to hear this high-pitched lung sound
- Basilar crackles – wet lung sounds heart at the base (bottom) of a lung (bibasilar crackles would be crackles over both lung bases). Crackles are also called rales
- Coarse rhonchi – low-pitched lung sound typically occurring in the upper airways (bronchi) due to bronchitis
- Inspiratory stridor – a high-pitched sound that is considered a sub-type of wheeze. It is caused by narrowing or obstruction of the upper airway (trachea or larynx) and is most often seen in croup, a condition only affecting children

Cardiovascular exam

Refers to examination by the doctor of the patient's heart and circulatory system. It usually consists of listening to the patient's heart in several locations and possibly checking pulses in any/all extremities (arms and legs). The unremarkable exam of the heart may include the terms below:

- Regular rate and rhythm (RRR) – rate refers to the heart rate, recorded as the number of beats per minute (bpm), typically 60-80 is normal. Rhythm refers to a consistent pattern/time interval between beats and a normal rhythm is called a "normal sinus rhythm" (NSR)
- No gallops, rubs or murmurs – no abnormal sounds. Typically the heart beat has two identifiable sounds ("lub-dub", called S1 and S2). Extra "lubs" or "dubs" are called a gallop and murmurs are whooshing sounds in-between the "lub-dub"

Pulses

The pulses may be checked at an annual physical exam or specifically in patients with diabetes or advanced age and who are at greater risk of vascular disease (blood vessel disease). In these patients, arterial blood flow may gradually slow and be noticeable on exam as a weakly palpable pulse. This can have serious implications, like gangrene and amputation, if left untreated. The major pulses that the physician may check include the:

- Dorsalis pedis (or pedal) pulse – on the top of the foot
- Posterior tibial (PT) pulse – behind the medial malleolus (bump) of each ankle
- Femoral pulse – in the groin
- Brachial pulse – in the inner upper arm, sometimes checked in children and infants
- Radial – just proximal to the wrist on the thumb side (radial aspect)
- Carotid – in the front of the neck

The measurement of the pulses, like many of the other scales used in the physical exam, is graded from 0 to 4+ as below:

- 0 – absent (not palpable)
- 1+ – diminished
- 2+ – normal
- 3+ – increased
- 4+ – bounding

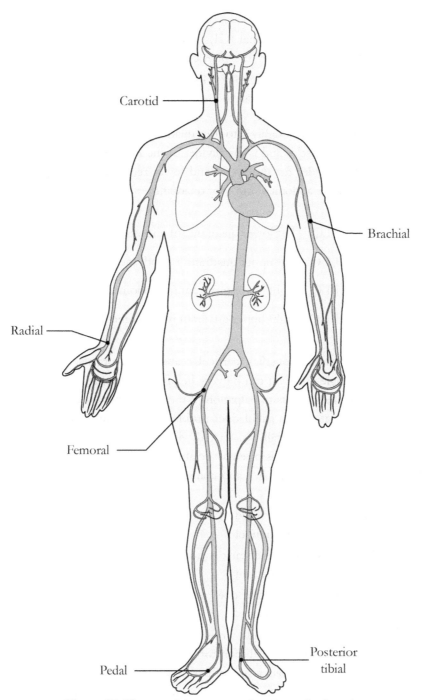

Figure 17: The arterial system and major pulse locations

Abdominal (GI) Exam

The abdominal or gastrointestinal (GI) exam includes examination of the patient's abdomen ("belly") by the physician. It is primarily examined via palpation, but may also be assessed via percussion (for tympanitic sounds) or auscultation (for bowel sounds).

The abdomen is divided roughly into four quadrants. The midline is formed by the abdominal muscles and is the divider of the left and right sides. The umbilicus is the divider for the upper and lower regions. These two lines effectively divide the abdomen into four quadrants:

LLQ   left lower quadrant (of abdomen)

LUQ   left upper quadrant (of abdomen)

RLQ   right lower quadrant (of abdomen)

RUQ   right upper quadrant (of abdomen)

Because each quadrant overlies particular abdominal organs, tenderness localized to a single quadrant can be very helpful in discerning the cause of a patient's pain. Tenderness to palpation of the right upper quadrant (RUQ) is generally associated with gallbladder problems; and right lower quadrant (RLQ) tenderness is classically associated with appendicitis; and left lower quadrant tenderness (LLQ) is often associated with diverticulitis and colitis. However, the unremarkable abdominal exam may include these components:

- **Soft** – in contrast to hard or firm, as when a patient is distended due to gas, constipation, etc.
- **Non-distended** – abdomen is not bulging outward (compared to the patient's usual anatomy).
- **Non-tender** – palpation does not cause discomfort in any of the four abdominal regions.
- **No rebound**– more fully known as rebound tenderness, rebound is a sign of increased discomfort when pressure is removed from part of the abdomen, a sign of peritonitis.
- **No guarding** – voluntary or involuntary flexion of the abdominal muscles during exam to prevent increased discomfort when

palpated.

- Bowel sounds normoactive – examined via auscultation of the abdomen, normal bowel sounds are in contrast to absent bowel sounds (as in regions distal to a bowel obstruction) or hyperactive bowel sounds (as in diarrhea from gastroenteritis). Many physicians do not listen for bowel sounds.

- Non-tympanitic – percussion (or tapping) on the abdomen produces consistent sounds throughout the abdomen. Hollow or tympanitic sounds are due to gas in the bowel.

- No hepatosplenomegaly – enlargement of the liver or spleen, which may occur with various diseases.

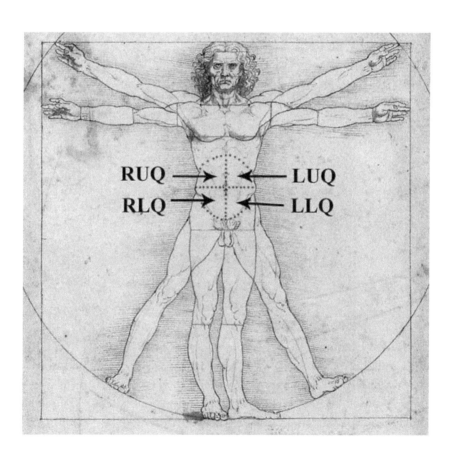

There are several other generally accepted regions of the abdomen that don't fall into the classic quadrant arrangement. The epigastric (gastric refers to the stomach) region is in the midline and above the umbilicus. The periumbilical region is around the umbilicus. The suprapubic area is just above the pubis (the anterior pelvic bone) and the flanks are the extreme sides of the abdomen.

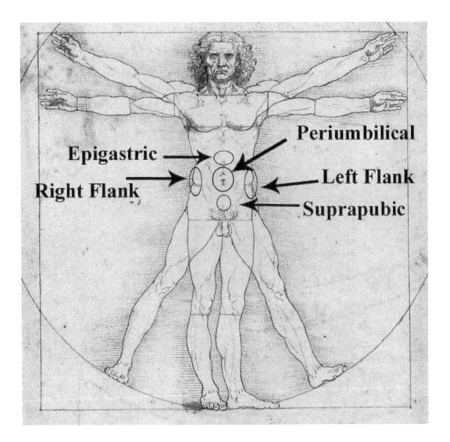

The Rectal Exam

The rectal exam is a part of the GI exam that is sometimes performed if there is concern about hemorrhoids or other external abnormality, or to obtain a stool sample for occult (hidden) blood analysis. The rectal examination consists of external inspection, followed by insertion of a single finger into the rectal vault called the digital exam. The finger can palpate internal hemorrhoids and other masses. If a patient is complaining of constipation or similar symptoms the physician may be able to palpate firm rectal stool and obtain a stool culture, if indicated. In male patients, the prostate can also be palpated via the rectum anteriorly. This is called the prostate exam, if it is performed.

- No evidence for fistula or fissure, no external hemorrhoids.
- No mass on digital exam.
- Normal appearing, occult-negative stool in rectal vault.
- Guaiac negative stool – the guaiac test uses a piece of paper covered in a compound that turns blue when hemoglobin is present in a stool sample.
- Normal, smooth prostate without significant tenderness to palpation.

Genitourinary (GU) Exam

The examination of the penis, scrotum and testicles constitutes the male genitourinary exam (see "Pelvic Exam" for the female-specific genitourinary exam). The scribe may be excused from the room for the genitourinary exam for the patient's privacy. The GU exam is often performed on younger children during well-child checks and the removal of the diaper and examination of the genitals and perineum are an important part of the pediatric skin exam. The GU exam may also be performed for adults with genital-specific complaints. Generally, this exam consists of inspection, and sometimes palpation of the scrotum and testes. Normal exam findings may include:

- Normal external genitalia.
- No scrotal swelling or tenderness to palpation of the testes – this may be a sign of an inguinal hernia, epididymitis (inflammation of epididymis), orchitis (testicular inflammation), or testicular torsion
- No blood at the urethral meatus.
- No genital lesions noted – this may be indicative of a sexually transmitted infection.

The Pelvic Exam

The genitourinary examination in women is called the pelvic exam. General external genitalia inspection is often the first step in the pelvic exam. Then more specifically the pelvic examination consists of a bimanual exam and a speculum exam. For the bimanual exam, the provider uses both hands to feel the patient's uterus, ovaries and adnexa (structures adjacent to the uterus, including the ovaries and fallopian tubes). One hand rakes downwards on the patient's lower abdomen and two fingers of the other hand are inserted into the vagina. Masses and other abnormalities can be felt with the hands. Another important part of the bimanual exam is evaluation for cervical motion tenderness (CMT). For this part of the exam the provider will move the patient's cervix with the fingers inside the vagina. The patient will experience extreme pain with the maneuver if CMT is present. This can be indicative of a pelvic infection. In the speculum exam, a metal or plastic speculum is inserted into the vagina so that the cervix can be visualized and samples can be obtained, if needed. A PAP smear is the collection of cervical cells and analysis of them underneath a microscope to look for dysplastic ("abnormal growth") cells that might suggest cervical cancer. The speculum exam also allows for inspection of the vaginal vault/walls. Normal exam findings may include:

- Normal external genitalia/vulva
- Physiologic vaginal discharge within vaginal vault
- No adnexal mass or tenderness noted
- No cervical motion tenderness

Breast Exam

The breast exam is performed annually for females greater than 30 years of age and is typically performed to look for early signs of breast cancer. It is especially important in patients that have had a first-degree relative with breast cancer. Normal findings may include:

- No palpable masses – any mass, especially one that is firm with discrete borders and is only present on a single side is suspicious
- No dimpling or erythema of the skin or nipple – again, some cancers cause skin breakdown of the nipple and areola and this is a concerning findings
- No nipple discharge – this may represent ductal cancer, though nipple discharge is a very non-specific symptom; bloody nipple discharge may occur normally during the third trimester of pregnancy
- Normal axillary nodes – the lymph nodes in the armpits (axillae) are the first location that breast cancer often spreads to and palpation is performed to look for unusual masses

Neurological Exam

Performed in more comprehensive physical exams such as patients who present with a problem that may be neurological (e.g., stroke, AMS). The unremarkable exam may include these and more terms:

- Alert – the patient responds to verbal and, if necessary, to painful stimuli.

- Oriented times three – the patient knows who they are (person), their place (building, town, etc.) and the time (date, month, or year). When combined with alert (above), it is written as A&O x 3.

- Cranial nerves II-XII intact – the cranial nerves are the 12 nerves that originate directly from the brain & brainstem (as opposed to spinal nerves which originate from the spinal cord). They're mainly involved in sensation/movement in the face/head and the special senses (e.g. taste, sight, hearing). The doctor will test the cranial nerves by having the patient perform numerous tasks (e.g. sticking out the tongue, frowning, raising eyebrows) and doing tests such as the pupil exam and extra-ocular movements. The nerves with sensory and or motor functions in the face appear to be working properly. This is done by asking the patient to smile, close their eyes, open their eyes wide (eyebrows up), and other simple commands.

- Motor and sensory function intact in all four extremities – the patient has normal strength and sensation in both arms and both legs. Strength is graded from 0 to 5 with 0/5 strength meaning the patient has no voluntary muscle contraction and 5/5 strength considered normal muscle strength. This can be checked by providing resistance against a particular movement. Sensation is checked by testing the patient's recognition of light touch and ability to differentiate between sharp and dull objects. In diabetic patients, monofilament testing may be performed to check the function in the toes, as diabetic neuropathy (nerve damage) can cause loss of sensation in the feet.

Reflexes

Reflexes are intact and symmetric – the reflexes checked are normal and equal to the opposite (contralateral) side (e.g. left and right patellar reflexes).

Reflexes are sometimes recorded on a scale of 0-4 listed below. For example: "2/4 bilateral patellar reflexes present" would represent normal patellar reflexes. The rating scale is as below:

0   Absent

1+   Diminished

2+   Normal

3+   Increased, but normal movement (no clonus)

4+   Markedly hyperactive with clonus (involuntary and repeated muscle contractions)

Common reflexes:

- Achilles Reflex – tapping of the Achilles tendon elicits contraction of the calf.
- Bicipital Reflex – tapping of the bicep muscle at its insertion near the antecubital fossa (the crease in the arm) elicits movement of the biceps muscle.
- Brachioradialis Reflex – tapping of the distal forearm elicits jerk of this muscle.
- Patellar Reflex – tapping the knee with a hammer or finger; elicits jerking of the leg.

Psychiatric Exam

Based mainly on the interview of the patient. If the patient is obviously agitated or having hallucinations at the time of the interview, these observations would fall under the heading of the psychiatric exam. Some terms encountered may include:

- Hallucinations – patient is seeing or hearing things that don't exist (auditory or visual hallucinations).
- Suicidal or homicidal ideation – patient has or does not have the intention of harming himself/herself or others.
- Affect – the range of emotions that a person displays. A flat affect would mean the patient displays very little emotion (happy or sad) and would be indicative of depression. A labile affect (displaying high range of emotions) would be suggestive of bipolar disorder.

Skin (or Integumentary) Exam

Can be complete or a partial exam of only exposed skin or a small region of the patient's skin. Often the skin exam focuses on a specific area when the patient has a skin-related chief complaint. Includes these terms:

- Abscess (subcutaneous) – a collection of pus beneath the epidermis.
- Abrasion – superficial skin wound; a scrape.
- Bruising (contusion) – a collection of blood beneath the skin (hematoma), typically due to trauma; does not blanch.
  - o Petechiae – small (1-2 mm) red spots due to minor capillary hemorrhage.
  - o Purpura – medium (3-10 mm) red or purple spots.
  - o Ecchymosis – large (> 10 mm) hematomas; a typical bruise.
- Cyanotic / cyanosis – the bluish / purplish discoloration of the skin due to low oxygen saturation ("cyan" is a type of blue).
- Erythema – redness
- Incision (surgical) – a clean, straight break in the skin (due to surgery).
- Induration – hardening and thickening of the skin due to inflammation; it often occurs surrounding an abscess.
- Fluctuance – palpable collection of fluid.
- Jaundice – yellow color due to liver dysfunction.
- Pale – as may been seen in patients that are anemic.
- Pruritic – itchy
- Rashes
  - o Macules – flat
  - o Papules – raised
- Ulcers – lesion in skin; skin breakdown.
- Urticaria – hives, typical for allergic reactions.
- Warmth – skin is warm to the touch (palpably warm).

Musculoskeletal Exam

Often brief unless the patient presents with a muscular problem. These terms may be listed in this section:

- Costovertebral angle (CVA) tenderness – the point where the ribs meet the spine in the back; tapping (percussion) on this region may induce pain in those with pyelonephritis or kidney stones.
- Crepitus – crackling or popping sounds heard beneath the skin, generally referring to abnormal joint sounds.
- Edema – swelling due to fluid leaking into a tissue; it may be noted in the "Extremity" section of the physical exam, if present. It may be called pitting edema and rated as 1+ (mild pitting edema) to 4+ (severe pitting edema).
- Effusion – accumulation of fluid within a body cavity (e.g. a joint effusion or pleural effusion).
- Obvious deformities – broken bones or dislocations, essentially.
- Range of motion (ROM) – the ability of a joint to move through various positions, depending on the joint.
- Spasm – involuntary contraction of a muscle, common after injury, especially in the low back.
- Sprain – ligament injury.
- Strain – muscle or tendon injury (remember the "t" for tendon)
- Tenderness – increased discomfort upon palpation

Additional Objective Data

The following sections of the medical note are also regarded as objective data. This includes lab studies, radiology studies, and EKGs. These materials will typically be ordered after the initial history and physical exam and will not be available when you are initially writing the medical note.

Laboratory Studies, "The Labs"

Blood tests are the most common type of lab because of the great variety of molecular markers that can be found in the blood, but lab results also include throat swabs (to look for strep throat), urinalysis (a urine analysis), and cultures of various body fluids (urine, stool, blood, sputum).

Radiology Studies

Radiology studies consists of x-rays, computed tomography (CT) scans, magnetic resonance imaging (MRI), and ultrasounds. The results of x-rays, CT scans, MRIs and ultrasounds should all be recorded in the medical record. Often these studies are reviewed by a radiologist and the formal "reading" is returned to the ordering physician, often electronically or by fax. There are many ways to describe a normal imaging study, some examples of these include:

- No acute disease
- No acute cardiopulmonary process – this may be used to describe a normal chest x-ray
- No acute intracranial process – this may be used to describe a normal head CT

In contrast, any abnormal study cannot be summarized with these very general words that we can use to describe a negative study. You should look for the radiology report and copy that into the patient's note, when applicable, or ask the physician to dictate their read to you.

Electrocardiograms (EKGs or ECGs)

EKGs are frequently obtained for patients who have chest pain, syncope (loss of consciousness) or who present for a pre-operative evaluation to make sure they are healthy enough for surgery.

EKGs will be interpreted by the physician and this reading will be placed into the medical record. With many EKG systems, a computer-generated report will be generated, though the physician must still review and the EKG and state whether they agree or disagree with the electronic reading. EKGs are a billable procedure in some facilities, so it is important that this is documented correctly. Three findings are typically necessary, even in the case of a normal EKG, to be able to bill for that EKG.

First, we will describe the basic characteristics of an EKG (don't worry, we won't get too technical). Then, we will include some examples of abnormal EKG findings.

An EKG is an electrical reading of the patient's cardiac conduction—the heart's electrical activity. Regular conduction produces an EKG that has a few key landmarks. These include the P-wave, QRS complex, and T-wave as shown below.

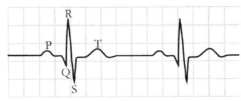

Figure 18: normal EKG

Describing a normal EKG like the one above will involve these basic variables:

- Normal sinus rhythm – this represents the normal conduction pattern of the heart, beginning at the sinus node. Interruptions in this usual conduction pathway are called "blocks," such as a right bundle branch block (RBBB), left bundle branch block (LBBB) or AV block.

- Normal axis – this simply refers to the baseline of the EKG (between T- and P-waves), which is typically flat without an incline or decline.

- Normal intervals – this refers to the time between the major points on the EKG. For example, the QRS interval is the time between the Q-wave and S-wave.

- As is discussed in Chapter 8, signs of a major heart attack occur between the S and T regions on an EKG. These are called ST changes, which may include an ST elevation or ST depression. Most "normal" EKG readings by the physician will explicitly state that there are no ST changes because of the serious nature of an ST change (heart attack).

Now that we've covered the most basic of EKG characteristics, a few examples are listed on the following page to help familiarize you with the format and terminology.

EKG (normal): Normal sinus rhythm, normal axis, normal intervals, normal QRS complex, no ST segment changes

EKG (abnormal; acute MI): Significant inferior and anterior ST segment elevation consistent with acute myocardial infarction. Normal sinus rhythm, normal intervals, normal QRS complex width.

EKG (abnormal A-fib): Irregularly, irregular rhythm consistent with atrial fibrillation, narrow QRS complex, diffuse non-specific ST segment changes.

EKG (abnormal; SV tachycardia): Initial EKG, 20:34: Supraventricular tachycardia, narrow complex, rate of over 200-210 beats per minute, no diagnostic ST segment changes.

Repeat EKG, 20:57: NSR with ventricular rate of 57, normal QRS, normal intervals, no ST segment abnormalities.

EKG: (abnormal): Sinus tachycardia with T wave inversion laterally and inferiorly. First degree AV block noted. Narrow QRS complex.

Again, you do not need to know how to read EKGs, but your physician may very likely dictate EKG findings to you, so you need to be able to recognize the terms that they mention and spell them correctly in the medical record.

Assessment and Plan (A&P)

The assessment and plan may be written together or separate depending on physician preference. Together, they will address the major complaints that the patient mentioned in the HPI. For example, if a patient feels very tired and is sleeping far more than previously, does the physician think the patient is depressed vs hypothyroidism? These parts of the note are the lone areas that the medical scribe cannot fully complete for the physician. If you are listening attentively while the physician interacts with the patient, you should be able to write in the A&P for the physician. You should change any "layman's" terms that the physician uses with the patient and use a slightly more medical term, when able. Nonetheless, despite your best efforts, the physician may need to add a few additional details based on their insight to the problem.

Frequently a problem list will be placed in the assessment or another part of the patient's note. This is often a simple list of the patient's past and present diagnoses. This is used as the foundation of the assessment and each problem may have a few sentences devoted to describing the physician's thoughts and treatment plan for that particular problem / condition.

The accuracy and detail in these sections is important per se, but they are also important for these reasons:

1. They outline the thoughts of the physician and are often reviewed by consultants or other physicians evaluating the patient.
2. The complexity of the assessment and plan is important for billing (to be discussed in Chapter 10).
3. High quality documentation can be very helpful from a medicolegal standpoint.

Below is an HPI from an annual physical exam (labeled as "Subjective" based on the SOAP note format) with the corresponding assessment and plan (A&P). Note that a well written medical note like the one below will have a logical flow from the HPI to the A&P (e.g. "She has right heel pain [HPI]... history and physical exam are completely consistent with plantar fasciitis [A&P]").

SUBJECTIVE: The patient is an X year old here today for the above. She has lost 10 lbs recently, about 1 lb per week, and is very happy about this. She has done this by increasing her activity and calorie restriction. The weight loss may have improved her blood pressure; when I saw her a year ago, it was borderline elevated at 152/98 and 147/89 on recheck. Today it is 126/81, which is great to see.

She has right heel pain that is worst right when she gets out of bed in the morning and when she walks after sitting for a few hours. As she moves around throughout the day it improves.

She is on methotrexate for psoriasis, and this gives her significant nausea.

She actually is fine with not completely clear skin but thinks her dermatologist is really trying to get it completely resolved. Dermatology also checks labs for methotrexate.

HEALTHCARE MAINTENANCE: She gets her eyes checked every 1-2 years and she wears glasses for driving. She has bilateral hearing aids, and they work well. Dental care is up to date and she goes every 6-12 months. From an immunization standpoint, she received a Tdap in 2012 and needs seasonal influenza immunization. Her last mammogram was in 2009 and she is due. Her last Pap was in 2009 as well. She has never had an abnormal Pap smear. She has been married for over 20 years and had been completely monogamous. She has no first-degree relatives with colon cancer, so screening for this will occur at age 50 for baseline purposes. She is fasting so will check a lipid panel and glucose.

ASSESSMENT AND PLAN:
1. Adult physical exam, up-to-date with health care maintenance strategies.
2. Seasonal influenza immunization given today.
3. Weight loss - it sounds like she is doing this in a healthy way and is happy about her results so far. Her blood pressure, which was borderline elevated one year ago, is great today at 126/81.
4. Right heel pain - history and physical exam are completely consistent with plantar fasciitis. We discussed that both stretches and heel inserts can help with the pain. I explained that stretches are especially important prior to the times when pain is worst - getting out of bed and after she has been sitting for a while.
5. Mammogram has been ordered.
6. Psoriasis - she follows closely with dermatology for this and feels it is under control. She has not really considered phototherapy yet and that might be a good option for her to discuss with her dermatologist given that she really does not like to be on things like methotrexate.

Diagnosis and ICD-10

The diagnosis or diagnoses are important because they summarize the reason for the patient's clinical visit very concisely. It essentially tells future readers what the doctor believes to be the underlying reason for the patient's symptoms. Often this is one of the first things seen in the note by physicians in other hospitals and clinics.

All diagnoses have an associated international classification of disease, 10th edition (ICD-10) code attached to them. Each digit or letter of this six-digit code provides information regarding the patient's diagnosis. These numbers are transform highly variable diagnosis into a list of numbers and are used for analysis by the Centers for Medicare and Medicaid Services (CMS), the body of the U.S. government that monitors these two services.

Review of the Medical Note

Once again, here is the general outline of the ED medical note. After reading this chapter you should have a much better understanding of each component of the note. Remember, the "SOAP" headings are not usually placed in the notes but are written to give you a mental framework of the organization of the note.

SUBJECTIVE:

Chief Complaint (CC)
History of Present Illness (HPI)
Review of Systems (ROS)
Allergies
Medications
Past Medical History (PMHx)
Past Surgical History (PSHx)
Family History (FHx)
Social History (SHx)

OBJECTIVE:

Physical Exam (PE)
Laboratory Results
Imaging Results

ASSESSMENT:

Diagnosis/Impression

PLAN:

Plan/Follow-Up
Discharge Medications

A Complete Note

You have officially read everything about the medical note! Below—to put everything together—is an example of a complete note, as documented by a medical scribe. For more examples, refer to Appendix A in the back of the book.

CC: Diabetic check

HPI: John Smith is a 47 yo male with a history of type II diabetes (diagnosed in 2011) and hypertension who presents for a diabetic check. He was last seen in clinic 6 months ago at which point his A1C was 8.1 and we started him on 500 mg BID metformin. He has been doing well since; no hospitalizations. He checks his blood sugar every morning before breakfast, typically around 105. He denies any polyphagia, polydipsia or weight changes. His last eye exam was 1 year ago and he is due for another, but he denies any visual changes. He denies any lower extremity paresthesias and no skin breakdown to note.

ROS:
Constitutional: No weight loss
Eyes: No vision changes
Cardiovascular: No chest pain
Neuro: No lower extremity paresthesias

Allergies: Penicillin (rash), peanuts (anaphylaxis)

Medications:
- ASA 325mg daily
- Metformin 500 mg BID
- Metoprolol 50 mg BID

Past Medical History: No previous records are available, but according the patient:
- Diabetes Mellitus, type II (diagnosed 2011)
- Hypertension
- Pneumonia 2009

Past Surgical History:
- Appendectomy 1982
- Right fibula fracture 1985
- Lasik, bilateral 2010 and 2011

Family History: Father has hypertension, alive. Mother has type II diabetes, alive. Sister has hypertension but is otherwise healthy.

Social History: Never smoked, occasional ETOH. Enjoys racquetball for exercise. Works at Wells Fargo.

Physical Exam:
Vital Signs: Heart Rate: 72, Respiratory Rate: 14, Blood Pressure: 133/84 Oximetry: 99% on room air Weight: 220 lbs (100kg)

GENERAL: Patient is pleasant, well groomed, well nourished, no acute distress

ENT: Normocephalic, atraumatic.

EYES: No conjunctival injection. PERRL, EOMI.

NECK: Supple.

RESPIRATORY: Lungs are CTA without rales or rhonchi. Good air movement.

CARDIOVASCULAR: Regular rate and rhythm. No murmurs, rubs or gallops. DP and PT are 2+ and symmetric.

NEUROLOGIC: Awake, alert and oriented x 3.

MONOFILAMENT: Intact sensory function in the feet bilaterally

PSYCHIATRIC: Normal affect, normal speech.

SKIN: Exposed skin is within normal limits. No ulceration or skin breakdown.

Laboratory Results
Basic Metabolic Panel:
Sodium   140   [135-145]
Potassium   4.9   [3.5-5.0]

Creatinine   1.0   [0.6-1.2]

Complete Blood Count:
WBC   7.8   [4.0-11.0]
Hgb   14.0   [12.0-17.0]
PLTs   370   [140-400]

Microalbumin to creatinine ratio   40   [30-300]

HgA1C   7.1

Imaging Results:
None

Assessment
1. Type II Diabetes Mellitus – well controlled with metformin. A1C improved from last visit. No evidence of neuropathy or nephropathy today. Continue 500 mg BID. Get eye exam soon. Follow-up in 6 months.
2. Hypertension – stable, continue metoprolol.

Plan
Follow up in 6 months. Continue current medication regimen.

SECTION 2:
FAMILY MEDICINE

5. THE PRIMARY CARE CLINIC

The clinic is an organized yet chaotic conglomeration of people. It mixes billing and administrative personnel, physicians and physician assistants, general practitioners and specialists, nurses and medical assistants. Despite its scheduled patient flow, it can be a fast-paced and disorganized center. To help familiarize you with the patient flow in the clinic, we will detail some of the major functions of clinical personnel below.

Registration and Medical Support Staff

- Registration – check patients into the clinic and verify their medical insurance
- Certified medical assistants (CMA) - place patients into rooms, obtain the chief complaint, record vitals, administer vaccinations, and perform simple tests like EKGs

Providers

- Nurse practitioners (NP) – nurses that have undergone graduate level training (doctor of nursing practice) that allows them to provide care, write prescriptions, etc. with or without the oversight of a physician.
- Physician assistants (PA-C or "PA") – care providers that function somewhat independently from an overseeing physician, but are required to have all treatment plans "signed off" by the specific physician with whom they work.
- Physicians – either medical doctors of allopathic (MD) or osteopathic (DO) medicine, they coordinate the care of specific patients and refer them to specialists, as needed.

Reviewing Patient Charts

Before the patient even sits down in their room, the doctor can know why they are coming into clinic, and it is your job to do so as well. You can do this by a few different means, which we will detail in the list below:

Prior encounters

The bulk of information about why the patient is presenting to clinic can be ascertained by looking at their last clinic note. Was that note nearly 1 year ago? If so, then they are likely arriving for an annual physical. It is helpful to look at the assessment from this prior encounter, as this may say when and why the patient was asked to follow up. For example, maybe their blood pressure was elevated at last visit and the doctor started them on an anti-hypertensive medication and they wanted to re-check their blood pressure 4-6 weeks later. You should be familiar with this process of reviewing old patient notes by the time you are working on your own as a scribe.

In addition, the physician may have ordered lab or imaging tests that need reviewing. These may not have been returned by the time that the last encounter finished. Or, in another scenario, the patient may have had the tests performed a few days prior to the current visit. In either case, the doctor will discuss the results and the implications of them at the current clinic visit. Hence, it is important to mention any tests ordered for a particular purpose (mammogram due to a new lump, chest x-ray because of an ongoing cough, etc.). These tests are in contrast to routine labs like a blood count (CBC), metabolic panel (BMP), or urinalysis (UA) and are ordered very frequently as a general screen.

Consult notes

Similar to the first method, it is important to review any and all notes since the last time the doctor saw the patient. This includes notes by other doctors, which are generally done via referral to a specialist. The specialist may perform testing and then refer the patient back to the primary physician for a more personal discussion about their medical care. It is important to know what the specialist thought (i.e. read the assessment from that encounter!) so that you are up-to-date when the patient arrives to clinic. To make sure you understand the different types of specialists, we have provided a brief summary of the different specialists below.

Cardiologist	Physician who cares for the patients with more complicated heart issues. Straight-forward cardiac conditions may be managed by the internist, but the cardiologist may be consulted on more complex issues. They may recommend specific cardiac testing or alter a patient's heart related medications.
Family practitioner	A general practitioner (GP) that focuses on routine medical care and preventative medicine in infants, children, adults and the elderly.
Gastroenterologist	Expert of the gastrointestinal (GI) system. They are consulted for patients with more diagnostically complicated GI system disorders (compared to something like appendicitis, which may simply be removed surgically). They may also perform endoscopies of the upper (EGD) or lower (colonoscopy) GI tract.
Hospitalist	Physicians, usually internists, who admit patients to the hospital and round on them throughout their stay. Family practice physicians and pediatricians can also sometimes fulfill the role of hospitalist.
Internist	Internal medicine physician that is an expert in adult medicine. They function in both the clinic and hospital settings. Hospitalists are often internists. This should not be confused with interns, who are first year residents.
Neurologist	An expert on nerve and brain disorders such as seizures, thromboembolic (clot) strokes, and other non-surgical issues.
Orthopedic surgeon (orthopedist)	Surgeon who cares for patients with bone problems or musculoskeletal injuries like a torn rotator cuff or ACL (of the knee).
Otolaryngologist (ENT)	Otolaryngologists are surgeons that strictly operate on the ears, nose and throat including surgeries like tympanostomy tubes, tonsillectomy, septoplasty, etc.
Pediatrician	Physician who takes care of children up to the age

	or 18 or 19. They may work in clinic and round within a hospital.
Surgeon	Physician who performs surgery. They may perform elective surgeries that require the patient to recuperate in the hospital or they may be consulted on more emergent cases like trauma or sepsis.

Recent hospitalizations

Recent hospitalizations, just like consults, are important to review prior to seeing the patient. We will discuss the common reasons for hospitalization in the following chapters, so it won't be elaborated on here.

6. ROUTINE PATIENT ENCOUNTERS

Patients may present to clinic for any number of reasons, but a large proportion of the visits fall into easily definable categories that are worth the time to understand. Some of these include the routine visits like annual physicals, well child checks, sports physicals and pre-operative visits. This chapter will describe the purpose of these visits and inform you of the typical diagnostics performed during each.

New Patient Visits

Patients that are new to a particular clinic often have an initial visit aptly named a "new patient visit." These visits are not meant to address a particular complaint (like knee pain), but are meant for the patient to "establish care" (these are the big keywords) with the provider. This means going over the patient's prior medical, surgical, family and social history and addressing the preventative screenings that are not up-to-date. Your job as a scribe is to make sure these various details are up-to-date in the electronic medical record for future visits. The various preventative screens will be detailed beneath the annual physicals header in this chapter, as they are often performed on a year-to-year basis.

Annual Physicals and Preventative Medicine

Patients typically try to see their doctor once every year, even if they are healthy, in order to maintain a relationship with their doctor. Thus, patients may not have any complaints during this visit and the medical note will therefore cover a lot of social history (as outlined in Chapter 4). It is important to capture this social information and keep it up-to-date for the next visit.

From the physician's perspective, the major goal of these visits is to make sure the patient is up-to-date on preventative screening. These tests are ordered every few years to identify early signs of disease, exactly how often depends on the test and the patient's risk factors. The most common preventative screens include those listed and described in the following paragraphs.

Pelvic Exam and PAP Smear

A pelvic exam is typically performed during every annual physical exam of a female patient over age 21. The pelvic exam includes two steps:

1. Cervical exam – using a speculum, the physician will examine the cervix and may perform a Pap smear of the cervical tissue. A Pap smear is the microscopic examination of the cervical tissue sample to look for signs of early cervical cancer called neoplasia or dysplasia ("plasia" means growth, hence these two terms mean "new growth" and "abnormal growth").

2. Bimanual exam – two fingers are inserted into the vagina up to the cervix and then pressure is applied from outside the abdominal wall onto the uterus. This looks for tenderness of the uterus and adjacent structures including the fallopian tubes and ovaries, which together are called the uteran adnexa. An adnexal mass may be the first sign of an ectopic pregnancy.

Mammogram

A mammogram is essentially an x-ray directed at the soft tissue of the breasts that looks for abnormally dense regions within the breast. These lumps or masses may be an early sign of breast cancer, one of the leading causes of death in women. The guidelines for mammogram screening vary depending on the organization, but generally screening begins between age 40 and 50 and is repeated every 1-2 years thereafter.

Colonoscopy / Flexible Sigmoidoscopy

These two tests are performed by a gastroenterologist to look for evidence of colon cancer. A flexible sigmoidoscopy is the use of an endoscope (a small fiberoptic camera) inserted in the rectum and going only up to the sigmoid colon (the S-bend in the left lower quadrant). A colonoscopy uses the same fiberoptic camera to examine the entire colon and typically require more preparation beforehand (e.g. no eating and lots of laxatives).

Again, the age at which colorectal cancer screening should begin varies depending on organization. For those without a family history of colorectal cancer, screening typically begins at age 50 and is repeated every 5 or 10 years. In people with a family history of colorectal cancer this may be started at age 40 and repeated more frequently.

DEXA Scan

DEXA (or DXA) stands for Dual-Energy X-ray Absorptiometry and is used to measure the bone density of those at risk for osteoporosis and osteopenia. Post-menopausal women are at greatest risk for bone mineral loss and screening typically begins around age 65.

This is a somewhat complicated scan with a lot of calculations performed, but the most important result is the overall T-score. The T-score is a comparison of the patient's bone density compared to a healthy 30 year old person. A negative T-score represents a loss of bone density. The important ranges for T-scores are:

- A T-score of <-2.5 is defined as osteoporosis ("porous bones")
- A T-score of -1.0 to -2.5 is defined as osteopenia ("reduced bone").

Patient's with osteopenia and osteoporosis will almost certainly be recommended to take daily calcium and vitamin D supplements to improve bone health. The next line of treatment is with a bisphosphonate medication that reduces the breakdown of bone, the most common medication being alendronate (Fosamax). Repeat testing is done after a minimum of 2 years as changes in bone density occur very slowly; Fosamax is typically only given for a total of 5 years during a person's lifetime because by inhibiting the cells that break down bone, it also impairs the body's ability to repair micro-fractures and may lead to pathologic (relatively atraumatic) fractures.

Prostate-Specific Antigen (PSA) Testing

PSA testing is performed to look for abnormally high levels of an antigen secreted by the prostate gland, a circular tissue surrounding the male urethra. It is a highly controversial test because it is very non-specific, meaning an elevated PSA does not necessarily indicate cancer. This is problematic because patient's with an elevated PSA might be put through a rigmarole of testing and even prostatectomy (removal or the prostate), which often has the side effect of urinary incontinence and erectile dysfunction. In addition, prostate cancer is nearly ubiquitous in males of advanced age and is often very slow to advance, hence there is a good chance it might not even progress to cause symptoms until after the patient would have died of another cause. This is not to say all forms of prostate cancer are slow growing and non-invasive, just that this non-hereditary, late-in-life form typically is this way.

Given all this controversy, PSA testing may be more likely to be performed in males with a particular indication for testing. This may include males with a family history of prostate cancer or in those with an abnormal prostate exam, which is palpated from within the rectum; an abnormal exam may include a palpably enlarged or irregularly shaped prostate gland. If performed, PSA testing it is usually started around age 50 and repeated every few years.

Testicular Exam

The testicular exam is a manual palpation of each testicle to assess for lumps that may indicate testicular cancer as well as bulges while coughing that may represent an inguinal (groin) hernia. This is a fairly straightforward examination and is performed for men of all ages. In fact, testicular cancer is unique in that its incidence peaks for men between 25-34, as can be seen in the chart below.

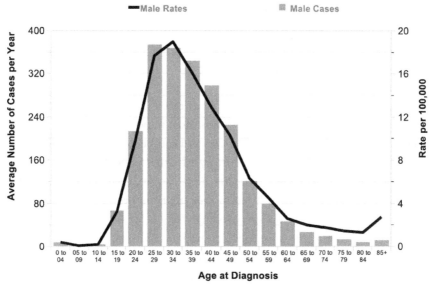

Source: http://info.cancerresearchuk.org/cancerstats/faqs/#How

Figure 19: Incidence of testicular cancer by age

Annual Physicals: Women

Beginning at age 21 women get an annual cervical exam to look for polyps (growths) due to cervical cancer. During the cervical exam, the physician may scrape off cells from the cervical wall, collect them, and send them off for microscopic analysis. This is a PAP smear and it is performed to look for abnormal cells that may be indicative of early cervical cancer. It is often performed every 3 years in women 21-30 years old. After age 30, women will still receive an annual cervical exam, but a PAP smear and HPV (human papilloma virus) testing will only be performed once every 5 years. HPV

Cervical cancer is one of the leading causes of death in women, but the single most deadly cause is breast cancer. For women, annual or biannual mammograms begin as early as age 40 or as late as age 50. This test uses low-energy x-rays (much like a CT scan) to detect changes in density within the breasts, such as a cancerous mass or calcification. Often times this test will be performed a few days prior to an office visit, as it takes a couple of days for the results to return.

Post-menopausal women (i.e. those that no longer experience menstrual periods, generally occurring in the late 40s or early 50s) are susceptible to increased rate of bone loss and will have a DEXA scan beginning around age 65.

Annual Physicals: Men

Beginning as early as age 45, men may start receiving a digital prostate exam to check for an enlarged prostate. This is most important for men that have a family history of early prostate cancer, and can be delayed until a later age for those without this family history. If the patient is experiencing symptoms of an enlarged prostate (e.g. poor urine flow, hesitancy, frequency, etc.) and/or the physician feels that the prostate is enlarged on palpation, then they may undergo testing to look for prostate cancer. This lab test is called the prostate specific antigen (PSA) test. The PSA test is controversial because prostate cancers are typically very slow to advance, and an elevated PSA may start a chain of events that include further testing and even removal of the prostate (prostatectomy), which may cause urinary incontinence or erectile dysfunction. This can significantly impair quality of life and may be completely unnecessary because an enlarged prostate does not mean it is cancerous. Many aging men have what is called Benign Prostatic Hyperplasia (BPH), which is a non-malignant enlargement of the prostate.

Well Child Checks (WCC)

Newborns

Neonates, or newborn babies, typically require follow up with their family physician 2-3 days after leaving the hospital. This is to make sure the baby is feeding adequately, to monitor healing of the circumcision in boys, and to observe for any jaundice. It is important to note the birth weight (e.g. 6 lbs, 15 oz), discharge weight (which is often slightly below birth weight since they don't feed immediately after birth), and Apgar score. The Apgar score quantifies the health of a newborn and is generally assessed 1 minutes and 5 minutes after birth.

Category	Score of 0 (min)	Score of 2 (max)
Appearance	diffusely cyanotic	no cyanosis
Pulse	absent	>100 bpm
Grimace/irritability	no response to stimulation	cries or pulls away when stimulated
Activity	None	Flexes arms and legs with resistance
Respiratory effort	Absent	Strong, lusty cry

Jaundice is a yellow discoloration of the skin and eyes due to elevated levels of bilirubin, a breakdown product of heme metabolism. While in the womb, bilirubin is processed by the mother's placenta. After birth, the baby's liver must start performing this function and often it takes a couple days to a couple weeks for the liver to become self-sufficient. Thus it is not uncommon for newborns to have some degree of jaundice, which usually is not problematic, but requires monitoring by the physician.

Infants and Toddlers

Well child checks for young children focus largely on the child's physical and mental development. The typical appointments occur at 2, 4, 6, 9, 12, 15, 18, and 24 months of age. Growth charts at these visits will track the infants increase in their height and weight compared to other infants of the same age. Ideally, a child should continue along a growth curve (percentile) and it is worrisome if a patient starts dropping in their percentile from one visit to the next. An example of a standard growth chart is pictured on the following page.

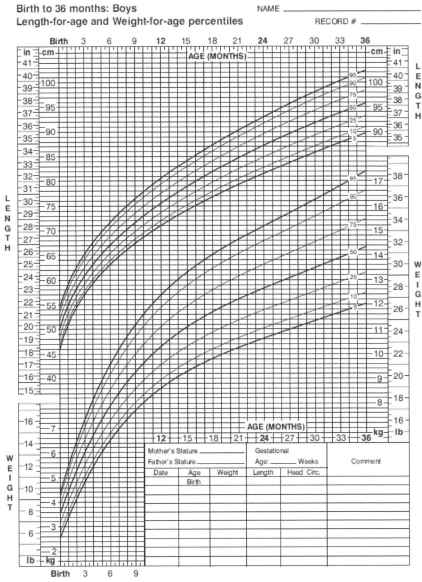

Figure 20: Growth chart for boys age 0-36 months. Source: CDC

The mental, emotional, and social development of the child is equally important. Together the appropriate steps in development in these categories are called "milestones." There are certain milestones that occur at each age (and at each well child check). The Centers for Disease Control and Prevention (CDC) lists 3-4 milestones at each age as seen below. Note, that because this is a checklist (for you and the physician), this is something that you do NOT have to memorize.

Age	Milestones
Birth	Recognizes caregiver's voice Turns head toward breast or bottle Communicates through body language, fussing or crying
1 Month	Starts to smile Raises head when on tummy Calms down when rocked, cradled or sung to
2 Months	Begins to smile at people Coos, makes gurgling sounds Begins to follow things with eyes Can hold head up
4 Months	Babbles with expression Likes to play with people Reaches for toy with one hand Brings hand to mouth
6 Months	Knows familiar faces Responds to own name Brings things to mouth Rolls over in both directions
12 Months	Cries when mom or dad leaves Says "mama" and "dada" Copies gestures (for example, waves "bye bye") May stand alone
15 Months	Imitates what you are doing Drinks from a cup Scribbles on his own Walks well
18 Months	Points to show others something interesting Says several single words Points to one body part May walk up steps and run

Vaccinations are also an important part about infant well child checks. The vaccination schedule is quite complex and recommendations change from time to time, so memorizing the exact guidelines is unimportant assuming that the physician has the checklist available. You should, however, be able to recognize the vaccinations in a medical note and in the conversation with the parents.

Hepatitis A & B	A viral infection affecting the liver
Rotavirus	a common cause of severe diarrhea in children
DTaP	Diphtheria, Tetanus and acellular Pertussis ("whooping cough").
Hib	Haemophilus influenza type b, a cause of meningitis and pneumonia in infants
Inactivated poliovirus	A viral infection that has been largely eradicated but was well known as the disease most likely causing president Franklin Delano Roosevelt's (FDR's) paraplegia
Influenza	The seasonal flu virus
Pneumococcal	Pneumonia
MMR	Measles, Mumps, Rubella
Varicella	Chicken pox

Sports Physicals

Sports physicals are typically performed for teenagers prior to participating in a competitive sport. Often these teenagers are high-school aged and generally healthy and therefore merely have to be checked over by the physician. This interaction will include a lot of general questions about the patient's health, like how much calcium do they intake every day, are they maintaining a stable weight, etc. This evaluation will also include a glance at the patient's growth chart to make sure they are maturing appropriately. The physician will likely perform a full physical exam during this encounter.

Pre-Op Visits

If a patient is undergoing a surgical procedure, the surgeon typically has the patient see their primary physician for a routine pre-operative visit. The tests performed during this visit will depend on the patient's medical history and the severity of the procedure they are undergoing. Patients with a prior cardiac history undergoing intermediate risk surgery as well as patients undergoing high risk surgery will receive an EKG. In addition, a CBC will often be ordered if significant blood loss is expected; patients taking anticoagulants (including fish oil and aspirin) will nearly always stop taking these medications prior to surgery to minimize blood loss. Further pre-operative testing will be dependent on the surgery (e.g. a urinalysis prior to a prostatectomy) and the patient's comorbidities (e.g. an A1C in a diabetic patient).

7. MANAGEMENT OF CHRONIC DISEASES

Many of the non-routine visits fall under the heading of disease management. There are a couple conditions, in particular, that represent a large proportion of these visits to clinic. The conditions that we will discuss in this chapter are not immediately life-threatening, but they increase a patient's future risk of a catastrophic event—like a heart attack or stroke. Therefore, the management of these conditions is a high priority for the family physician. It is not important for you to understand every theoretical facet of these visits, but we hope that by providing you with more detailed information about these few conditions that it will improve your abilities as a scribe.

Type II Diabetes Mellitus

There are two types of diabetes mellitus: Type I and Type II. Type I diabetes is an autoimmune disorder that results in the destruction of the β-cells of the pancreatic islets, which normally produce insulin. Insulin is a hormone that signals cells throughout the body, especially the cells of the liver that store and regulate glycogen (a long-chain sugar), to take up and store blood glucose. This is especially important after eating when the carbohydrates found in foods like grains (breads, pastas, etc.) and sweets are broken down into individual sugar molecules (called monosaccharides); when this happens, blood glucose rises. Because an elevated blood glucose can have dangerous immediate and long-term effects, insulin helps to lower blood glucose and prevent these outcomes.

Type I diabetics, because they do not produce insulin, must receive exogenous (from outside the body) insulin to control blood glucose levels. Type II diabetes is an acquired condition rather than an autoimmune condition. It represents the vast majority of all cases of diabetes and is the reason that it is the primary type that we will explain in this chapter.

Type II diabetes results from an insensitivity to the usual effects of insulin. This means that when a person with type II diabetes eats a carbohydrate-rich meal, the cells of the body respond with less vigor to insulin. As a result, blood glucose levels remain high after eating.

Diagnosis of Type II Diabetes Mellitus

The diagnosis of type II diabetes is fairly straightforward. In patients without type II diabetes screening labs like a basic metabolic panel are obtained every 3-5 years. In patients with other comorbidities, like hypertension, an annual physical exam may also include a basic metabolic panel. This set of labs includes a blood glucose. If a patient's blood glucose is abnormal on one of these screening tests, then more definitive labs are ordered. The first, may be a fasting glucose. Fasting means that this lab is done when the patient has not eaten in several hours, typically overnight; this reflects the lowest level of a person's blood glucose. An abnormal result is called an "impaired fasting glucose" and can be a sign of pre-diabetes or diabetes altogether. Ultimately, there is one lab that is used to diagnose and monitor diabetes: the hemoglobin A1C. Hemoglobin is a molecule found in red blood cells and is necessary for oxygen transport. Irreversible glycosylation (binding of sugar) can occur at the end of the hemoglobin molecule; when it does, the resulting molecule is called hemoglobin A1C (because it binds to an *alpha* amino acid). A higher blood glucose throughout the lifetime of a hemoglobin molecule, the more glycosylated it becomes. Because red blood cells (and their hemoglobin) typically circulate for 120 days before broken down, the hemoglobin A1C lab test is used as an estimate of the average blood glucose over a period of 3-4 months. The table below shows the ranges for hemoglobin A1C values and the cutoff for normal, pre-diabetes, and a diagnosis of type II diabetes.

	A1C Level (%)
Normal	< 6.0
Pre-diabetes	6.0-6.4
Diabetes	≥ 6.5

Management and Monitoring of Type II Diabetes

Once a patient has been diagnosed with diabetes, a patient may require medical management and more frequent monitoring.

The decision on whether to start a patient on a medication for type II diabetes depends on the level of their A1C. A1C values are used for more than just the diagnosis of diabetes, but they are used to monitor it as well.

As you can see in the following table, A1C levels are directly correlated to average blood glucose levels.

A1C level (%)	Average Blood Glucose Level (mg/dL)
5	90
6	120
7	150
8	180
9	210

Because A1C levels can inform you about the relative severity of a patient's type II diabetes, they can be used to influence treatment decisions. The first decision, is this: does a patient need a medication or can they simply control their diabetes by altering their diet? The latter of these is called diet-controlled type II diabetes and represents a more mild form of diabetes. If a patient fails to take control of their blood glucose on diet alone, then a medication will be necessary. The medical management of diabetes follows this basic 3 step progression:

First Line Medication: Metformin
Metformin is the safest of the blood glucose regulators. It decreases serum glucose by sensitizing the patient's body to circulating insulin. Because it does not affect the amount of insulin circulating in the body, it poses very minimal risk for hypoglycemia, which may occur with the second and third line medications. For these reasons, metformin is the near-universal first-line choice for the management of type II diabetes. Of note, because metformin is excreted by the kidneys, it should not be used in patients with chronic kidney disease (Cr $\geq$ 1.5) because these patients may fail to filter the medication from the bloodstream.

Second Line Medications: Insulin Secretagogues
Insulin secretagogues are the second-line medications for the treatment of type II diabetes. These medications stimulate the secretion of insulin from β-cells (and inhibit glucagon release) and can be used instead of (not with) prandial insulin products. You do not necessarily have to remember the names of specific medications, but there are common features to the names of the medications, as you can see:

- Glimepiride
- Glipizide
- Glyburide

Third Line Medications: Insulin products

If a patient fails to control their blood glucose levels on the first and second line medications, then he/she may require injectable insulin to further control their blood sugar. There are two primary categories of insulin products based on whether they are slow- or fast-acting.

Basal insulin products are slow-acting and provide an insulin baseline throughout the day. They typically last 12 hours and therefore may be taken twice a day—once in the morning and once at night. The most common brand of basal insulin is Lantus.

Prandial insulin products are fast-acting and are typically taken around mealtime to counteract spikes in blood sugar. They are added to a basal insulin regimen when high volumes of basal insulin are required to control blood sugar. The most common brand name prandial insulins include Humalog and NovoLog.

Although there are some medications that are fast or slow acting, there are many intermediate forms and some that even include a combination of both types.

Complications of Type II Diabetes

We already mentioned the hemoglobin A1C and its utility in monitoring a patient's diabetic control, but there is more to a diabetic clinic visit that just this lab. The high blood sugars associated with diabetes cause a lot of vascular (i.e. blood vessel) damage throughout the body. There are a few regions of the body with very small blood vessels that are especially sensitive to the inflammatory damage caused by diabetes; hence they are dubbed the "microvascular" complications of diabetes. The three microvascular complications of diabetes are known by the three **P**s.

- Neuro**p**athy
- Nephro**p**athy
- Retino**p**athy

Neuropathy is the loss of sensation and/or motor function due to damage to a nerve. This often occurs in the feet and legs because of poor blood flow. When it presents as a loss of sensation, it predisposes the patient to skin ulcers, especially in the feet. This may occur because of tight-fitting shoes or anything that rubs against the feet. The loss of sensation prevents the patient from recognizing the skin breakdown, resulting in significant skin ulceration before they notice the damage. Diabetic neuropathy, being one of the common microvascular complications of diabetes, is examined by yearly foot exams and monofilament testing. To test the sensory function of the foot, the physician uses a thin filament called a monofilament. Essentially, monofilaments are thin rods of material that buckle at pressures above a certain threshold. This occurs when the doctor puts the end of the filament against a specific region of the foot (see image below) and pushes until the monofilament bends. This directs a precise amount of pressure into the patient's foot and in a non-diabetic would be felt as pressure. In patients with diabetic neuropathy, they may not be able to sense the minor amount of pressure caused by the monofilament and this would be an early sign of diabetic neuropathy.

Diabetic Foot Screen Sites

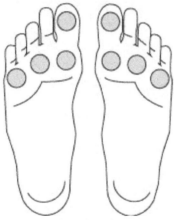

Figure 21: Sensory testing sites for the diabetic foot exam

Diabetic nephropathy is kidney damage stemming from long-standing diabetes mellitus ("*Neph*" refers to the nephron, the functional unit of the kidney). The root cause is damage to the glomerular capsule, the filter and first part of the nephron (also known as Bowman's capsule). This capsule is porous and allows ions and other small molecules into the nephron whilst large molecules like proteins bypass the kidneys altogether. The damage to the glomerular capsule that occurs with diabetes results in larger pores in the filter, allowing molecules like proteins to enter the kidneys and eventually into urine. To test for early diabetic nephropathy, a lab called a microalbumin is ordered. This looks for microscopic levels of albumin, a ubiquitous protein found in the bloodstream, in a urine sample. The test is positive if albumin is present in the urine, which means that a large protein has inappropriately slipped through the glomerulus. The most precise test is the microalbumin to creatinine ratio (ACR), which compares the amount of microalbumin to creatinine in the urine. Diabetic nephropathy is defined as an ACR of > 30 mcg per milligram of creatinine, but the values are less important than simply understanding the rationale for ordering it.

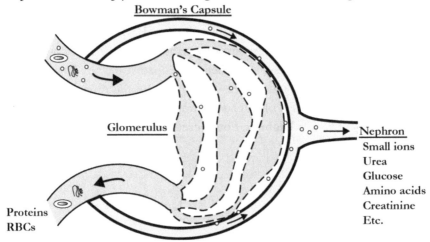

Figure 22: The glomerulus without diabetic nephropathy

Lastly, diabetes predisposes a person to retinopathy, a disease affecting the small blood vessels within the eye. The retina is the innermost part of the eye that is stimulated by light and is ultimately responsible for our vision. The blood vessels supplying the cells of the retina are especially sensitive to the inflammation associated with recurrent hyperglycemia. Through multiple postulated theories, the walls of retinal capillaries become weak and porous. Gradually, capillaries may narrow to the point that the cells of the retina receive a reduced supply of blood, causing cell death. While this is gradually occurring, the weakness of the capillaries increases the risk of macular edema: swelling in the region responsible for our highest acuity vision, resulting in blurred vision. All-in-all, diabetic retinopathy is the primary cause of new onset blindness in adults. Given all of this, diabetic patients require annual eye exams with an ophthalmologist (eye doctor) to check for early stages of diabetic retinopathy and other eye conditions that are also more common in patients with diabetes.

In conclusion, type II diabetes mellitus is the primary type of diabetes managed by the primary care provider. It is caused by an insensitivity of a person's body to the usual effects of insulin, which typically notifies cells to take-up glucose from the bloodstream. When cells are insensitive to insulin, blood glucose remains high after eating and this high blood glucose causes inflammation within a person's blood vessels. The blood vessels of the legs, kidneys, and eyes are the most sensitive to recurrent hyperglycemia and, when damaged, may result in diabetic neuropathy, nephropathy or retinopathy. The hemoglobin A1C blood test is the primary tool for the diagnosis and monitoring of type II diabetes mellitus. If necessary, patients with type II diabetes may require medications to improve their diabetic control and prevent the consequences (the three P's) of uncontrolled diabetes. Metformin is the universal first-line medication to control diabetes because it sensitizes the body to insulin. Second-line medications are the insulin secretagogues, which stimulate the secretion of insulin from the pancreas. And finally, patients that fail to control their blood sugar with these medications may require exogenous basal ("baseline") or prandial (mealtime) insulin.

Hypertension

Hypertension, or high blood pressure, is a vascular disease that—like diabetes—predisposes a person to more serious conditions in the future, if uncontrolled. Hence, patients with high blood pressure are regularly and routinely seen in the primary care clinic.

The management of hypertension, unlike most other conditions, is unique because it attempts to regulate a vital sign: blood pressure. Blood pressure is measured in units of millimeters of mercury (mmHg) and a "normal" blood pressure is defined as approximately 120/80 (read as 120 over 80). The first number indicates the systolic blood pressure; this is the maximum pressure against the heart when it is contracting. This number is highly variable and increases with exercise (and anxiety) to accommodate the demands of exercise. In this setting, high blood pressure allows for more rapid delivery of blood to the working organs according to this equation:

$$A_1 \times v_1 = A_2 \times v_2$$

Where A = cross-sectional area of a blood vessel and v = the velocity of blood flow. According to this equation, constricting a blood vessel (decreasing area of A_2) increases the velocity of blood flow (v_2). During exercise, the increased velocity of blood flow supplies the working muscles with a greater quantity of oxygen.

The second number of 120/80 is the diastolic pressure. This is the peripheral resistance against the heart in between heartbeats (when the heart is relaxed) and represents the minimum blood pressure; unlike systolic pressure, the diastolic pressure has minimal variability.

If normal blood pressure is around 120/80, hypertension, in contrast, is defined as a consistent blood pressure of greater than or equal to 140/90. To better understand the negative effects of high blood pressure, we need to look at what high blood pressure represents.

Blood pressure is an indirect measure of peripheral resistance. High blood pressure is damaging because greater resistance places greater strain on the heart to pump blood. To control blood pressure, there are several different classes of medications that can be used to lower blood pressure. Many of these medications act as vasodilators; these medications dilate or expand blood vessels. To see why this lowers blood pressure, you need to know the correlation between resistance and blood vessel radius:

$$R \propto \frac{L \times \eta}{r^4}$$

Where R = resistance, L = length of the vessel, η = viscosity of blood flow, and r = vessel radius.

You can see from this correlation that small changes in the radius of an artery (or the arterial system as a whole) can result in significant changes in resistance (e.g. a slight increase in vessel radius will cause a more significant decrease in resistance). This is why many of the anti-hypertensive medications are vasodilators.

Like diabetes, hypertension can predispose a person to diseases of particular organs that are sensitive to the reduced blood flow associated with hypertension. Acutely elevated blood pressure in the range of 220/110 can cause "end-organ damage." This means that certain organs receive so little blood flow because of severely narrowed arteries that cells of these organs actually die off. The organs of interest include the brain, heart, and kidneys—all of which may experience some degree of cell death as a result of severely elevated blood pressure and may result in a stroke, heart attack or renal failure.

Mildly elevated blood pressure, however, is not immediately worrisome. But if blood pressure is chronically untreated or undertreated, the gradual narrowing of the arteries to these same organs (brain, heart, kidneys) can increase the risk of a stroke, heart attack, and chronic kidney disease. For this reason, patients with hypertension require regular monitoring to ensure that the possibility of these conditions is minimized.

Monitoring Blood Pressure
Because hypertension is defined as an *average* blood pressure of greater than or equal to 140/90, there are a couple different ways to diagnose and monitor it. First, the patient should be seated comfortably for 5 minutes to make sure a blood pressure reading represents resting blood pressure, not

the elevated blood pressure that occurs with activity. At least two separate blood pressure readings on separate clinic visits are required for the diagnosis of hypertension. Some people have what is called "white coat hypertension" in which their blood pressure is elevated in clinic because of some underlying anxiety. All patients, but these patients in particular, may be asked to record their blood pressure at home in between clinic visits to obtain a better estimate of their average blood pressure.

Treatment of Hypertension

If a person's average blood pressure meets criteria for hypertension they may be started on a medication to reduce their blood pressure. If this occurs at one visit, the patient will require follow-up within 2-6 weeks to evaluate its effectiveness.

Many of the medications used to treat hypertension act as vasodilators, which decrease blood pressure according to the previously shown equation. However, there are several other medications that are classified as diuretics. Diuretics increase the rate of urine formation, thereby reducing the amount of water in the bloodstream. This decreases the total volume of blood. So rather than altering the radius of the arteries, diuretics decrease blood volume and thereby decrease the pressure within the arteries.

Although some of the medications produce the same end-result (vasodilation), they do so via different mechanisms. This is essential because high doses of a single medication may cause serious side effects; for this reason, each medication has a "maximum dosage" that should not be exceeded. Because of the maximum dosage set for each medication, a patient with persistent hypertension while on one of these medications may require a second medication from another class—not necessarily a higher dose of the first medication—to further lower blood pressure. The medications listed here are the most commonly used anti-hypertensive medications:

- Amlodipine (Norvasc)—a calcium channel blocker
- Hydralazine
- Hydrochlorothiazide—a thiazide diuretic. This medication increases the excretion of potassium. Therefore annual metabolic panels are required to monitor potassium levels

- Lisinopril—an ACE inhibitor
- Losartan—angiotension receptor blocker (ARB)
- Metoprolol, atenolol, carvidelol—beta blockers
- Triamterene—potassium-sparing diuretic often found in combination with hydrochlorothiazide

In summary, hypertension is the condition of having consistently elevated blood pressure, defined as greater than or equal to 140/90 mmHg. High blood pressure increases the resistance against the heart while pumping blood, and over the course of a lifetime, elevated blood pressure may increase the risk of heart failure. Blood pressure is typically correlated to the radius of blood vessels throughout the arterial system and high blood pressure is a sign of narrowed blood vessels. Uncontrolled high blood pressure is not immediately concerning unless it is in the range of 220/110, but the long-term effects of uncontrolled high blood pressure include an increased risk of a future heart attack, stroke, or renal failure. The treatment of hypertension includes medications that either increase the radius of arteries (vasodilators like beta-blockers and calcium channel blockers) or decrease blood volume (diuretics like hydrochlorothiazide and triamterene).

Hyperlipidemia

Hyperlipidemia, based on the word roots, is the condition of having high blood lipids. Typically this refers to abnormally high levels of low-density lipoprotein (LDL), a risk factor for atherosclerosis (formation of plaque within the arteries). However, a LDL level is only one of four components of the lipid panel and there are separate diagnoses for abnormal values of each component. Here are the four major components of a lipid panel, the range of normal, and the names of the conditions when a particular component is abnormal:

	Range (mg/dL)	Condition, if out of stated range
Total cholesterol	< 200	Hypercholesterolemia
LDL	< 100	Hyperlipidemia
HDL	> 40	Dyslipidemia
Triglycerides	< 150	Hypertriglyceridemia

To better understand these values we will outline each component in more detail.

Cholesterol

Cholesterol is an essential component of cell membranes and is synthesized at various sites in the human body. It is largely non-polar (hydrophobic) and thus is very ineffectively transported in the blood, which is largely composed of water (hydrophilic). Lipids carry cholesterol to and from the liver to cells that require it.

Low-Density Lipoproteins (LDL)

Because cholesterol is unable to transport itself through the bloodstream, a carrier molecule is required to transport it from the site of synthesis (e.g. the liver) to cells that require it. Low-density lipoproteins facilitate this transport to cells that express the LDL receptor. However, when LDL levels become elevated, some LDL molecules leak out without gaining their own LDL receptor. These LDL particles are phagocytized by macrophages, which die and deposit in the walls of the arteries; this is the formation of plague known as atherosclerosis. Because of this, high LDL levels are considered the major risk factor for cardiovascular disease.

High Density Lipoproteins (HDL)

High density lipoproteins have the opposite effect of low density lipoproteins. High density lipoproteins are the "good" cholesterol (even though they are not a cholesterol) and are considered cardioprotective. It is theorized that HDL molecules can remove LDL embedded in the walls of the blood vessels and transport it back to the liver. This is why low HDL levels are bad and it is optimal to have an HDL level greater than 40 mg/dL.

Triglycerides

Triglycerides are carrier molecules for fatty acids with each triglyceride containing three fatty acids. Triglycerides are unique because they are absorbed differently in the small intestine by the lymphatic system and transported directly into the bloodstream (instead of going directly to the liver like most nutrients). Triglycerides, like the other lipid panel components, are transported through the blood via a lipoprotein molecule. This lipoprotein molecule, when cleaved to release free fatty acids (the energy in triglycerides), can form atherosclerotic plaque just like LDL does. So high levels of triglycerides is another risk factor for cardiovascular disease.

Treating Hyperlipidemia, Etc.

There is a single class of medications (statins) used to treat hyperlipidemia and related conditions, but there are several other supplements that have some evidence to suggest that they too can improve an abnormal lipid profile. Many of these show some degree of activity with multiple components in the lipid panel, so for that reason we will discuss them as a whole:

1. Statins – statins inhibit the enzyme (HMG-COA reductase) that is responsible for the irreversible, rate-limiting step in cholesterol synthesis. Most statins are conveniently named so that the generic name includes the word "statin" within it (e.g. atorvastatin, simvastatin).
2. Niacin – as a supplement, niacin can lower LDL and increase

HDL.

3. Red Yeast Rice Extract (RYRE) – this supplement has the same pharmacologic compound as statins but is available without a prescription.

4. Fibrates – these medications are used in conjunction to statins to improve lipid profiles as a whole. The most common ones include fenofibrate (Tricor) and gemfibrozil (Lopid).

5. Fish oil – fish oils high in omega-3 fatty acids have been shown to be helpful in lowering triglyceride levels (hypertriglyceridemia).

Monitoring Hyperlipidemia

Changes in a person's lipid profile occur very gradually, so repeat lipid panels are obtained after at least 3 months of initiating statin therapy. However, a follow up lipid panel may not be repeated for 6 to 12 months for more mild hyperlipidemia.

In summary, lipids, cholesterol and triglycerides are molecules found within the bloodstream that can contribute to the formation of plaque within the arterial system. Hyperlipidemia is the condition of having elevated levels of low-density lipoprotein (LDL), which poses the greatest risk for atherosclerosis and depending on the blood vessels effected, may increase the risk of a heart attack or stroke. However, hypercholesterolemia (high cholesterol), dyslipidemia (low HDL), and hypertriglyceridemia (high triglycerides) also increase the risk of atherosclerosis. Statins are the most common medication used to decrease a patient's LDL level and many of the statin medications have easy to notice names like simvastatin (Zocor) and atorvastatin (Lipitor). Red yeast rice extract is available over-the-counter and may also decrease a patient's LDL through the same mechanism. Niacin, fibrates (e.g. fenofibrate) and fish oil may also improve a patient's lipid profile.

Hypothyroidism

Hypothyroidism is the condition in which the thyroid is underactive, as the name suggests ("hypo" means low). The thyroid is located immediately below and to the sides of the Adam's Apple, technically known as the thyroid cartilage. Thyroid hormone is produced in the thyroid and is actually composed to two separate hormones called T_3 and T_4, based on the number of iodine atoms found in each molecule. Iodine deficiency used to be the cause of goiter, a type of hypothyroidism, before the invention of iodinated salt. Modern hypothyroidism often occurs as a result of aging as the thyroid's ability to produce thyroid hormone diminishes; it is especially common in women over age 60. A simple blood test can be used to diagnose hypothyroidism. This tests for levels of thyroid stimulating hormone (TSH), a hormone created and secreted by the anterior pituitary gland. Paradoxically, because we are not directly testing thyroid hormone, but the hormone that stimulates it, a **low TSH** indicates that the thyroid is **over**active and a **high TSH** indicates that the thyroid is **under**active.

To understand this you need to understand the relationship between the pituitary, TSH, the thyroid, and thyroid hormone. This process is pictured on the following page. It begins when the hypothalamus (located in the brain, not pictured) secretes thyroid releasing hormone (TRH), which stimulates the anterior pituitary to release thyroid stimulating hormone (TSH). TSH then induces the thyroid to make more thyroid hormone (T_3 and T_4), which acts throughout the body and controls our basal metabolic rate. But T_3 and T_4 also exert negative feedback on the pituitary. That means that when levels of thyroid hormone are high, the pituitary is inhibited from producing TSH and TSH levels thereby decrease. Vice versa, when thyroid hormone levels are low, there is very little negative feedback on the pituitary and as such TSH levels become elevated. So a high TSH indicates that there is very little circulating T_3 and T_4 and hence a **high TSH is indicative of hypothyroidism.**

Because the thyroid hormones control our metabolic rate, patients with hypothyroidism may report symptoms of fatigue, unexplained weight gain, thinning hair, and depression. Treatment, however, is very simple. Patients will be prescribed a synthetic form of thyroid hormone, which goes by the name levothyroxine (Synthroid).

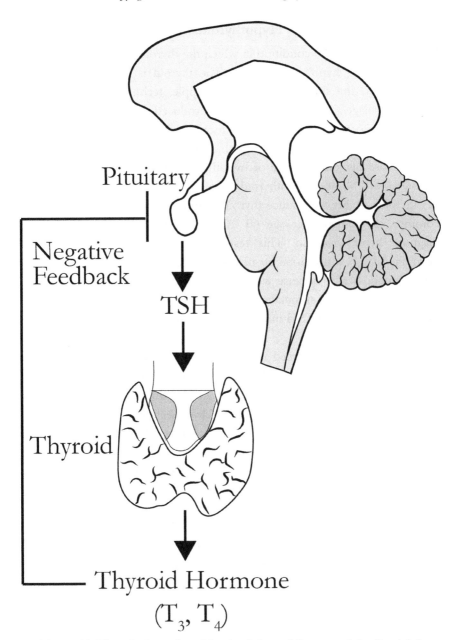

Figure 23: The pituitary-thyroid axis. Adapted from work by Patrick J. Lynch, medical illustrator; C. Carl Jaffe, MD, cardiologist.

8. UNDERSTANDING ACUTE MEDICAL CARE

Although you will be working in the primary clinic, not in the emergency department (ED), you will be seeing several patients after they visit the ED, urgent care, and/or are admitted to the hospital due to acute processes. As such, you will need to know the thought processes of an ED physician and the basic medicine accompanying these acute medical issues. This chapter will introduce the most fundamental knowledge of emergency medicine.

The emergency room is open 24 hours a day, 7 days a week, 52 weeks a year. ED physicians are tasked with evaluating patients that come in with a variety of complaints and thus act as a type of general practitioner. They see all types of people and problems and seek to answer one question: is this patient at significant risk for decompensation if they are discharged home? While it seems overly simple, this is the ultimate goal of emergency medicine: to act as a filter, sorting out the patients requiring admission and/or specialized care (e.g. surgery) from those patients that are safe enough to return home and follow up with their primary care physicians.

This approach to medicine can be thought of as the "rule out" method. An emergency physician does not necessarily try to diagnose the exact cause of a patient's symptoms (and often they do not, as a diagnosis may not exist or may be labor intensive to identify), but at the minimum he/she strives to identify the conditions that pose significant risk to the patient. For example, in a patient with chest pain there are a few conditions that will be on the forefront on the physician's mind including myocardial infarction (heart attack), pneumothorax, pneumonia, aortic dissection, and pulmonary embolism. The "workup" (i.e. all of the labs, imaging studies, and other tests performed in the ED) will therefore be focused on making sure that the patient's chest pain is not due to a serious underlying issue. Thus, as is true for patients with chest pain and various other complaints, it is essential to know the basic features of the "rule out differential" so as to better understand the physician's workup, interventions (like medications) and overall mindset as well. This is not strictly limited to the ED physician, as a patient with features suggestive of an MI or PE may also worry the primary care physician to perform certain tests.

You may think that it is unnecessary to understand these "rule out" conditions as a scribe. After all, the job description states that we as scribes listen to the interaction between the physician and the patient and document accordingly. Therefore, because the doctor is guiding the conversation and asking certain questions, is it really necessary to understand why particular questions are being asked? Of course! You may not have to memorize all of the minor details and ask the questions for yourself, but understanding the differential diagnoses will greatly improve your writing of the HPI. A truly great HPI demonstrates flow of thought. That is, the details of the HPI are arranged in such a way that the differential diagnosis is nearly self-evident. For example, in a patient with chest pain, the details may be written in such a way to suggest that the cause is a myocardial infarction rather than a pulmonary embolism. The workup for these two conditions may be quite different, so the HPI should foreshadow the workup that is to come. Essentially, the ideal medical note is one where an experienced practitioner can understand each step of the ED physician's thought process as they read each part of the medical note, beginning with the HPI and moving to the physical exam, workup, and eventually to the medical decision making. It is for this reason—the flow of thought in both the HPI and the note as a whole—that understanding the major "rule out" conditions is absolutely essential to writing a good note. The following sections will address the major "rule out" conditions for some of the most common complaints.

Chest Pain Differential

Chest pain is one of the most common complaints for patients presenting to the ED. The cause might be one of several worrisome conditions (MI, aortic pathology, pneumothorax, PE etc.), or it might be from muscle or tendon irritation (e.g. costochondritis), anxiety (which often causes chest "tightness," not pain), or any number of other causes. As mentioned above, the two of the somewhat common and worrisome conditions that cause chest pain are myocardial infarctions (MIs) and pulmonary embolisms (PEs). Each one typically causes slightly different types of chest pain and different associated symptoms. Given that chest pain is so common in the ED, understanding these differences is a critical skill for the ED scribe, as you will be writing innumerable chest pain HPIs. The following paragraphs will detail the pathophysiology, signs, symptoms and tests that differentiate between these two conditions. A table summarizing the signs and symptoms can be found at the end of this section and should, at the minimum, be what you take away from this section.

Acute Myocardial Infarction (a.k.a. Heart Attack)
A heart attack is a serious medical condition in which an artery supplying the heart muscle (coronary artery) is too narrow to provide sufficient blood flow to the heart. This causes impaired oxygen delivery to the heart, reducing its ability to contract and eventually causing cardiac cell death.

Any condition that causes arterial narrowing will predispose a person to a myocardial infarction, including hypertension (a.k.a. high blood pressure), which is often due to narrow arteries, and hyperlipidemia ("high lipids"), which is nearly synonymous with hypercholesteremia ("high cholesterol") and increases the likelihood of plaque formation within the artery.[1] This narrowing process occurs over a period of many years. Once an artery becomes narrowed by greater than 70% (more technically called >70% stenosis), then a patient may experience chest pain only with exercise (stable angina) for a period of days to weeks. This occurs because exercise raises blood pressure and causes vasoconstriction (arterial narrowing), which may further reduce blood flow in someone with an already narrowed artery and induce cardiac related chest pain. If the stenosis is more severe (> 90%), blood flow may be so limited that a patient experiences chest pain at rest (unstable angina). Once this occurs, the pain is often constant, though may improve with rest or medications that cause arterial vasodilation (nitroglycerin is the most common one and you should make sure to remember it!).

This cardiac related chest pain is typically located over the left chest and is described as a pressure-like pain (e.g. crushing or elephant on the chest). The patient may also experience diaphoresis, or excessive sweating, caused in response to shock as a result of the reduced cardiac output that occurs during a heart attack.

Women sometimes do not present with the classical left sided chest pain that men do. Symptoms like pain or discomfort in the left neck, jaw or arm are called referred pain, as the pain is felt at a site away from the original injury (the heart or left chest). One theory is that this may be due to a convergence of cardiac sensory neurons and neurons of the left arm and neck, which may confuse the brain into thinking the pain is coming from one of these other body regions. Regardless of the mechanism, a female with left neck, jaw or arm pain may be evaluated to rule out a heart attack as if they were experiencing chest pain. In addition, even in males with left chest pain, the physician may often ask if the pain radiates to the left arm, neck or jaw—hint, they're probing for symptoms that might suggest that the patient is having an MI.

Once the history is taken from the patient and it shows signs worrisome for a myocardial infarction, then the diagnostic workup begins. Patients will first get an EKG to look for changes in the electrical conduction of the heart. Large areas of cardiac death will no longer conduct electricity in the normal fashion and this "detour" in the conduction pathway can be seen on an EKG. The most recognizable type of "detour" is a change in the region between the S and T waves on an EKG and these changes are called an ST elevation or ST depression; they indicate a very serious myocardial infarction. As a scribe, you will not need to read an EKG and diagnose a heart attack, but just know that ED physicians typically look at an EKG specifically to make sure there are no ST changes. See the two EKGs on the following page and notice the differences between the normal EKG and the STEMI pattern.

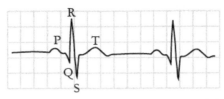

Figure 24: Normal EKG with P wave representing atrial depolarization (i.e. contraction), the QRS complex representing ventricular depolarization and the T wave representing ventricular repolarization (i.e. relaxation).

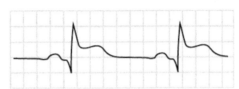

Figure 25: An ST-elevation myocardial infarction (STEMI), as evidenced by the raised axis or baseline of the wave pattern between the S and T waves.

After the EKG, a patient will have a lab test that looks for cardiac cell death. This test is the troponin I test. Troponin is a molecule involved in the contraction of muscle fibers and troponin I is specific for cardiac muscle. When cardiac muscle cells die, they release this troponin I into the blood, which can be tested in the lab. This release of troponin into the blood takes 3-6 hours after the initial injury and patients may often need repeat troponin I tests over a period of hours to be sure that a patient is not having a heart attack. This is called "serial troponins," and the patient may have these performed in the ED or they may be admitted to the hospital overnight to monitor these results.

Finally, if the EKG and/or the troponin I is abnormal a patient may need emergent cardiac surgery to either open the blocked artery or to bypass it. This is called cardiac catheterization, as a small catheter is inserted into the femoral or radial artery and guided into the heart. Fluorescent dye is pushed through the catheter into the coronary arteries and then hit with x-rays to create an image of the artery. When a stenotic artery is identified, blood flow may be restored via either stenting, which use metal supports to expand the artery), or bypass grafting (a.k.a. coronary artery bypass grafting; CABG), which removes a vein from the leg and uses it to create a detour around the coronary artery blockage.

Even if the workup is negative for a heart attack some patients with multiple risk factors (hypertension, hyperlipidemia, etc.) will still be admitted to the hospital for further monitoring and evaluation. Upon admission the patient will often be placed on telemetry, which is continuous monitoring of a patient's EKG. If the serial troponins, EKG, and telemetry are all normal, then a patient may undergo stress testing to evaluate for the risk of a heart attack in the near future. The most common type of stress test takes images of a patient's heart before and again after strenuous exercise and looks for changes in function. This is called a stress echocardiogram. A negative stress test has a very high negative predictive value over the next year, meaning that a normal stress echocardiogram suggests that the patient will not have a cardiac event in the short-term.

Now how does this translate into writing an HPI? We hope this information will help you summarize important information from patients that are following up after an emergency department visit and/or hospitalization. For example, if you are following-up on a patient that was admitted for left sided chest pain/pressure 2 days ago, well now you should have the knowledge to write this: "Two days ago he was admitted with left sided chest pressure and had a negative workup including an EKG, serial troponins, chest x-ray, and stress echo."

That is a fairly detailed summary of the signs, symptoms and tests to evaluate for a heart attack. Next, we will overview the basics of evaluating for a pulmonary embolism, which actually is quite similar—pathophysiologically—to a heart attack—except that it affects a lung.

[1] Note that the other 3 risk factors for heart disease include: diabetes mellitus, smoking, and a family history of an early cardiac event (direct relative, such as a mother, father, brother or sister with a myocardial infarction before age 55 for men or before age 65 for women). These risk factors are very important for determining the likelihood that the patient is or will experience a cardiac event and it is always good to mention all 5 risk factors in a HPI for chest pain.

Pulmonary Embolism

In contrast to the slowly developing plaque formation that causes a heart attack, a pulmonary embolism occurs suddenly. By definition, it is the formation of an embolus (a clot that breaks away and travels in the blood stream to another site) and becomes lodged in an artery supplying the lung(s). We will first discuss the pathophysiology of embolization, followed by the signs, risk factors and tests used to diagnose a PE.

The prerequisite for a pulmonary embolism is firstly the presence of a thrombus. A thrombus is a clot that has NOT broken away and traveled through the blood stream, but instead remains where it is formed. Once this clot breaks away it is called an embolus, and the process of breaking away is called embolization.

Often, the site of thrombus (clot) formation is in the deep veins of the legs, though it could occur anywhere. This is called deep vein thrombosis (DVT). It occurs due to two primary processes: 1) Injury, such as trauma or surgery, which causes internal bleeding (or bruising) and promotes formation of blood clots to staunch the bleeding; and 2) Slow venous blood flow. Blood often pools in the legs due to the effects of gravity if sitting or standing for long periods of time. And when blood flow slows, it is more likely to clot. That is why long distance travel like international flights are notorious for causing blood clots; any similarly long periods of immobility therefore will increase the risk for DVT.

Now that we have established what causes DVT, we must explain how this leads to a pulmonary embolism. Once the thrombus has formed, it may dislodge and travel through the venous system to one of the venae cavaes (likely the inferior vena cava) and enter the right atrium. From there it enters the right ventricle and is pumped out to the pulmonary circulation. The clot now encounters small blood vessels for the first time and is sufficiently large to obstruct blood flow. The lodging of an embolus in the lungs is called pulmonary embolization (and the condition is known as a pulmonary embolism). Embolization can cause two problems:
1. Because blood flow from the heart is no longer reaching the lungs for gas exchange (respiration), the patient may become hypoxic (low oxygen, with the prefix "hypo" meaning low and suffix "oxia" referring to oxygen). Thus, hypoxia and sudden shortness of breath are common signs of a PE
2. Just as the blockage of a coronary artery causes cardiac cell death,

blockage of a pulmonary artery can cause pulmonary (or lung) tissue death. This too will contribute to hypoxia as the lung tissue itself becomes incapable of participating in respiration. The death and disintegration of lung tissue may lead to the tell-tale sign of a PE: hemoptysis (coughing up blood). Hemoptysis is a very specific symptom for a pulmonary embolism and is an important one to remember for the chest pain HPI.

To reiterate, pain associated with a pulmonary embolism typically begins quite quickly and is associated with severe shortness of breath. Depending on the lung and lobe affected, the location of the pain may vary (right or left sided, medial or lateral, etc.). The pain is often pleuritic as well. "Pleuritic" comes from "pleuritis" or inflammation of the pleura, which are the linings covering the lungs and thoracic cavity. If the pleura are inflamed, they often produce pain when they rub against each other, which typically occurs with deep inspirations. Therefore—in this long-winded explanation—pleuritic chest pain is pain that worsens with deep inspirations. This word is great because it gives you a one word description of chest pain for the first sentence of the HPI (the topic sentence), though you may still want to elaborate on the patient's specific description of the pain later in the HPI.

We have discussed the risk factors for clotting and the mechanism by which the clot lodges in a pulmonary artery. We now move to the diagnosis of a PE. The first step specifically undertaken to look for a PE is a blood test called a d-dimer; we say "specifically" because the patient may be getting tests for a heart attack as well, which you now know. Clots are made up of large cross-linked fibrous proteins made of fibrin. The body has enzymes that degrade these fibrin clots by cutting them into 2 unit molecules called dimers and one product is specifically called a d-dimer. Testing a patient's blood for the d-dimer molecule will evaluate for the presence of clots, though not specifically for a PE (it could be represent a DVT as well). If the d-dimer is positive, an ultrasound of the deep veins of the affected leg will be performed to look for DVT. If the ultrasound is positive for DVT, then a CT angiogram (CTA) of the lungs may be performed to look for clots within the pulmonary arteries ("angio" refers to blood vessels). If the CTA is positive for a PE, then medication will be administered to help degrade the clot, typically the choice is IV heparin.

Now that you know, in detail, the signs and symptoms of a heart attack and pulmonary embolism we want to make sure you remember the most pivotal details. The table on the following page summarizes the key differences between the two conditions. This should serve as the bare minimum of your knowledge of the chest pain differential, though we hope you retained some of the additional detail from the previous paragraphs.

	Myocardial infarction	Pulmonary embolism
Onset	Gradual	Sudden
Provoking factors	Exercise	Deep inspirations
Palliating factors	Rest, nitroglycerin	None
Quality	Pressure	Sharp
Radiation	Left neck, jaw, arm	None
Severity	10/10	10/10
Timing	Constant	Constant
Associated symptoms	Diaphoresis	Hypoxia, tachypnea

Summary table comparing MIs to PEs

We have focused on MI and PE, but other life-threatening causes of chest pain also often have very characteristic histories. For example, a spontaneous pneumothorax displays similar characteristics to PE. Aortic dissection will often present with severe, "tearing" chest pain that radiates into the back or neck. A patient with severe pneumonia will also frequently have severe associated pleuritic chest pain.

Strokes and Intracranial Hemorrhage

Strokes and traumatic intracranial hemorrhage represent the two most worrisome causes of acute neurological deficits. Typically, patients will present with a focal deficit like unilateral (one-sided) weakness, visual loss, difficulty speaking (called either expressive or receptive aphasia), or confusion. Because most regions of the brain have a very specific function, a patient may present with only a single discernible deficit (like garbled speech) rather than several deficits (like visual loss, lack of coordination, and aphasia).

Strokes

A stroke is the interruption of blood supply to the brain. This deprives brain cells of oxygen and can result in tissue death. Typically a stroke will cause a loss of neurological function (motor and/or sensory loss) in one side of the body in a contralateral fashion (e.g. a right sided stroke will cause neurological deficits on the left). The two causes of strokes are ischemia and hemorrhage. Hemorrhagic strokes are cases of intracranial bleeding, typically caused by the rupture of a fragile intracranial blood vessel like an aneurysm. Long-standing hypertension (a.k.a. high blood pressure), may contribute to the formation of these weak spots in a blood vessel and increase the risk for a hemorrhagic stroke. Ischemic strokes are more subtle and thus require greater historical detail to evaluate. The risk factors for an ischemic stroke depend on the type of stroke, either embolic or thrombotic.

Remember that a pulmonary embolism is caused by the formation of a clot within the leg that travels to the lung to obstruct pulmonary blood flow. This is nearly always the result when the clot forms in the peripheral circulation and travels back towards the heart. In contrast, when a clot forms in the heart itself it will be ejected from the heart back to the systemic circulation. When the destination is the brain, this causes an embolic stroke.

This may seem like an uncommon occurrence, but there is one very common condition that increases the risk of clotting within the heart itself—atrial fibrillation. Atrial fibrillation, or afib, is an irregularly irregular heart rhythm localized to the atria alone (not involving the ventricles).

Although the ventricles are more important to overall cardiac function (hence why ventricular fibrillation is life-threatening and afib is not), ventricular function is closely tied to atrial function since the atria fill with blood during diastole and transfer that blood into the ventricle for pumping. When the atria contract in a random, uncoordinated, and untimed rhythm—as in afib—it impairs the ability of the atria to fill and transfer blood to the ventricles. In addition, blood may "sit" or reside in a stagnant manner in the atria for a longer period of time because of the dyscoordination. And if you remember from our discussion of PEs, anytime blood flow slows (e.g. in the legs from long distance travel), it is more likely to clot. So afib increases the risk of clot formation within the heart itself. If a clot dislodges from the heart and is pumped out to an artery supplying the brain, an ischemic stroke may result. In summary, remember that afib is a HUGE risk factor for an embolic stroke! Because of this, patients with chronic or recurrent afib are placed on an anticoagulant ("blood thinner") like warfarin (Coumadin) to reduce the probability of blood clots and stroke.

In contrast to embolic strokes, thrombotic strokes are more common in the elderly and occur by the slower, more gradual mechanism of artery disease that was discussed in the section about myocardial infarctions above. However, to reiterate, the formation of plaque within an artery often occurs over a period of many years and hence why this is more typically confined to the elderly population. When this stenosis (or narrowing) occurs in an artery supplying the brain, a thrombotic stroke may occur. The risk factors for a thrombotic stroke include hypertension and hyperlipidemia (which also increase the risk for an MI), as well as a family history of stroke.

In patients presenting with neurological symptoms worrisome for a stroke, the physical exam will be heavily focused on the neurological section. Discussing this entire exam section is unnecessary in this chapter as it was previously addressed, but remember the sign of a stroke often includes a focal neurological deficit (unilateral weakness, visual loss, difficulty speaking, confusion, etc.).

Intracranial Hemorrhage (ICH)

Now although not technically considered a stroke, traumatic intracranial bleeds—including subarachnoid (SAH), subdural (SDH), and epidural hemorrhage—are also important to mention. The presence of blood within the confined space of the cranium, as may occur with a hemorrhagic stroke or an intracranial bleed (they are not synonymous), will compress the brain tissue and may cause focal neurological symptoms. In cases of acute head trauma, the physician will look for signs of a skull fracture, which may damage the blood vessels beneath the skull and cause a brain bleed. Raccoon eyes, which is essentially dark purple bruising beneath the eyes, is one example. Battle's sign, which is bruising behind the ear, is another sign of a skull fracture. Lastly, the physician may check the patient's ears for a hemotympanum, or blood behind the ear drum. The pooling of blood at any of these sites is indicative of a fracture of a particular cranial bone, which is beyond our scope here.

The exam for an ischemic stroke is more general and varied, with no particular test being highly specific to an ischemic stroke like the three signs above are for an intracranial bleed.

In summary, remember that there are two types of strokes (hemorrhagic, ischemic) and two types of ischemic strokes (embolic, thrombotic). In addition, there are two types of brain bleeds—hemorrhagic strokes due to an underlying vascular defect and intracranial bleeding secondary to trauma. You should remember the basic risk factors for each type of ischemic stroke, as patients with altered mental status or sudden onset of one-sided weakness / numbness will often be worked-up for a possible stroke. This means that the physician will almost certainly ask questions about many of these risk factors and will look for particular exam findings. Understanding what they are looking for will make you far more prepared as a scribe and an aspiring medical professional.

	Embolic Stroke	Thrombotic Stroke	Hemorrhagic Stroke	Intracranial hemorrhage
Etiology	Embolus (cardiac)	Thrombus	Aneurysm AVM	Head trauma
Risk factors	Afib	Hypertension Hyperlipidemia Family history	Hypertension Anticoagulation	NA
Physical exam findings	Unilateral motor weakness or sensory loss Slurred speech (dysarthria) Loss of language (aphasia)			Battle's sign Raccoon eyes Hemotympanum
Treatment	Aspirin Tissue plasminogen activator (TPA) ("clot buster")		Treat underlying cause and relieve brain pressure	Relieve brain pressure

Risk factors, physical exam findings, and treatment of strokes

9. SYSTEM-BASED MEDICINE

At this point, you understand type II diabetes mellitus, hypertension, hyperlipidemia, myocardial infarctions, pulmonary embolisms, and strokes. However, there are still several conditions that may be acute or chronic and are regularly seen by the primary care physician. We have organized these conditions by body system (e.g. respiratory system) and recommend that you familiarize yourself with the basics of each. The conditions described in this chapter include:

- Coronary artery disease (CAD)
- Atrial fibrillation (Afib)
- Congestive heart failure (CHF)
- Colitis
- Constipation
- Diverticulitis
- Gastroesophageal reflux disease (GERD)
- Peptic ulcer disease (PUD)
- Asthma
- Bronchitis
- Chronic obstructive pulmonary disease (COPD)
- Obstructive sleep apnea (OSA)
- Pneumonia
- Osteoarthritis (OA)
- Bursitis, sprains, meniscal injuries and strains
- Benign prostatic hyperplasia (BPH)
- Urinary tract infections (UTIs) and pyelonephritis

Although this may seem like a long list, this is quite concise in the scheme of all possible diseases of the various body systems. Write yourself notes about each condition on a separate piece of paper and carry it with you when you begin your clinical training. This will be a valuable resource when you encounter patients with one of these conditions.

Diseases of the Cardiovascular System

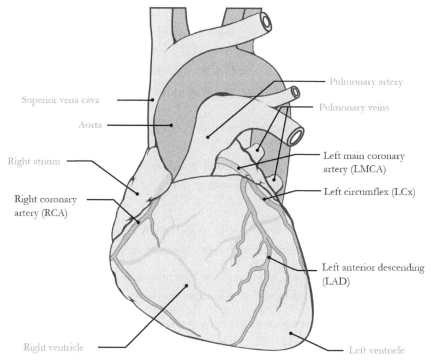

Figure 26: The human heart. Note the major coronary arteries including the notorious LAD, known as "The Widowmaker." This piece was originally created by Patrick J. Lynch, medical illustrator and adapted by Mikael Häggström.

Coronary Artery Disease (CAD)

Coronary artery disease, also called coronary heart disease, is a very common problem that affects a large percentage of the world's population. CAD is the buildup of plaques (atherosclerosis) in the arteries that supply oxygen to the heart. This can be problematic because the rupture of a plaque can lead to acute clot formation and blockage of the flow of blood to a portion of the heart. This event is called a myocardial infarction (MI) or "heart attack." A heart attack can be fatal or lead to substantial complications like congestive heart failure (CHF). CAD is the number one killer of men and women in the United States. Aggressive treatment and counseling of patients with this problem can substantially change the likelihood of near-term death in those effected. The primary care physician will often make medication and lifestyle management of these patients a high priority.

CAD is often completely silent, without symptoms, until it is too late. Some individuals with long-standing CAD will display chest pain on exertion or with stress. This is called angina and is typical in nature—it is sub-sternal, pressure-like and may radiate into the neck or arm.

Management of CAD focuses on the modification of established risk factors for the disorder.

1. Diabetes mellitus – maintaining good blood sugar control in these patients via lifestyle modification, and the use of oral medications and/or insulin.

2. Hypertension – maintaining good blood pressure control via lifestyle modification and the use of medications.

3. Hyperlipidemia – improved lipid profile through diet and lifestyle modification and the use of lipid-lowering medications.

4. Smoking – cessation of smoking is the single greatest way to reduce a patient's CAD risk. The use of counseling and sometimes medications is common.

5. Early family history of CAD – this can't be changed, but awareness is very important for the patient. Early family history of CAD is defined as a cardiac event prior to the age of 55 in men and 65 in women. This applies to a direct relative (i.e a sibling or parent).

Atrial fibrillation (Afib)

Atrial fibrillation is an irregularly irregular heart rhythm, meaning that there is no pattern to the irregular rhythm. It results from the atypical generation of electrical signals within an atrium rather than the sinoatrial node, which generates the normal (sinus) rhythm. These signals are generated so frequently that rather than contracting, relaxing, and then contracting again, the atria fibrillates. Fibrillation is the weak, rapid contraction of a muscle; you can think of fibrillation as "twitching" rather than "contracting."

Atrial fibrillation may be chronic or paroxysmal, meaning it may be constant or it may arise suddenly for short bouts, respectively. Atrial fibrillation is not immediately life-threatening, but it can cause symptoms like light-headedness or syncope. Ventricular fibrillation, in contrast is life-threatening because the ventricles, and specifically the left ventricle, are the most significant chambers when it comes to overall cardiac output.

When the atria contract weakly and out-of-sync with the ventricles, the transfer of blood from the atria to the ventricles is impaired. As a result, ventricular filling is reduced, which then limits the amount of blood pumped out to the rest of the body. This poor cardiac output may cause symptoms like light-headedness, orthostatic hypotension (low blood pressure upon standing), syncope/near-syncope, fatigue, and palpitations.

Afib not only causes decreased cardiac output, but there are additional side effects from turbulent cardiac blood flow as the atria fibrillate. When blood stagnates due to turbulent flow, it tends to form clots. As a result, while in afib, a patient's risk for clotting (hypercoagulation) increases significantly. Given this risk, patients with chronic or recurrent afib are prophylactically placed on chronic anticoagulants to minimize the risk of blood clots (e.g. Coumadin).

It should be noted that it is important that patients with new-onset afib, with a clear time of onset, be aggressively managed if they have not been in afib for more than 48 hours. If the patient can be moved back into normal sinus rhythm prior to 48 hours duration of afib, the risk of stroke can be mitigated to some degree. Often times these patients will be admitted to hospital and either medications or electricity will be used to convert the atrial fibrillation back to a normal rhythm. Once 48 hours have passed, the risk for stroke increases and anticoagulants and a more extensive workup will be necessary.

Congestive Heart Failure (CHF)
Heart failure may be an acute or chronic condition that is marked by an inability of the heart to provide an adequate supply of blood to bodily tissues. Chronic CHF results in a progressive deterioration in heart function, commonly secondary to advanced age and underlying disease

(hypertension, smoking, etc.).

One of the most characteristic signs of chronic CHF is an accumulation of fluid within the ankles, called lower extremity edema. Patients may also experience respiratory symptoms due to the accumulation of fluid in the lungs, such as orthopnea (dyspnea lying down).

Though not often checked in clinic, an elevated brain natriuretic peptide (BNP), a compound released in response to excessive ventricular stretching associated with fluid overload, is very suggestive of CHF.

The treatment of chronic CHF includes use of a diuretic to help expel the accumulated fluid. The most common type is called furosemide (Lasix). Because this fluid accumulation causes high blood pressure, patients may also be put on an ACE inhibitor like lisinopril or a beta blocker like metoprolol. Since these are three different types of medications, a patient may be prescribed all three of them.

Summary of treatment options:
1. Diuretic (e.g. Lasix)
2. ACE inhibitor (e.g. lisinopril), if necessary.
3. Beta blocker (e.g. metoprolol), if necessary.

Diseases of the Gastrointestinal (GI) System

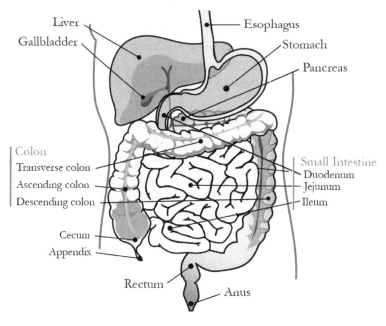

Figure 27: Overview of the gastrointestinal tract.

Colitis

Breakdown the word colitis and you will see that it means inflammation of the colon ("-itis" refers to inflammation and "col-" refers to the colon). Inflammation is a general word that should not be confused with infection; colitis could be caused by an infection, which causes inflammation, but the colon may be inflamed due to an immune system disorder and not an infection (e.g. "ulcerative colitis"). Nonetheless, infectious colitis is the most frequently encountered type of colitis. In this scenario, an infectious agent (generally bacteria) attack the wall of the colon, causing inflammation and pain in a fairly localized region. The most common sites are the sigmoid colon (the S-shaped bend in the left groin) or at the sharp turns in the bowel near the liver or spleen; these turns are called the hepatic and splenic flexures, respectively). Patients afflicted with colitis will often have a fever, elevated WBC, localized pain and innumerable episodes of diarrhea. A physician will be concerned about C.diff colitis, a particularly nasty type of bacterium (*Clostridium difficile*) that happens to cause particularly foul smelling stool. The inflammation of the colon wall can be seen on an abdominal CT as intestinal wall thickening. C.diff is the most likely cause of a newly diagnosed colitis, but exact identification requires a stool sample. If a stool sample is positive for C.diff, then patients will typically be treated with oral metronidazole (Flagyl) and ciprofloxacin (Cipro). Untreated colitis may result in perforation of the bowel as the bacteria eat through the intestinal wall and may be life-threatening.

Constipation

This is the most common cause of abdominal pain in children. It is characterized by infrequent stools or the passage of small, hard, pebble-like stools. Prune juice can be snuck into an infant's or toddler's food to help relieve it or the more formal use of medications like stool softeners (Miralax) or laxatives can be used for older children.

Diverticulitis

Diverticulitis is similar to colitis in that, as the name suggests, it involves inflammation, but it occurs at particular pouches or protrusions in the colon called diverticula (*singular* diverticulum) rather than along the length of the colon. These outpocketings form gradually during the aging process as the bowel wall weakens. The formation of these outpocketings is called diverticulosis and is commonly thought to be due to a low fiber diet that causes a person to strain excessively while defecating, which increases pressure within the intestines; however, this has not been proven. Regardless of the cause, these outpocketings in the colon wall tend to form in the sigmoid colon and they may trap fecal matter as it passes through the colon and hide them from the normal peristaltic waves that eliminate feces. The hidden fecal matter serves as a substrate for bacterial growth, which proliferates in this pocket and eventually starts attacking the wall of colon in this very localized region. Because the infection and inflammation is generally more localized than colitis, patients will often present with less pain and may not have a fever or elevated WBC. The diagnosis of diverticulitis is made by an abdominal CT, which will see a diverticulum (i.e. the outpocketing) with wall thickening (a sign of inflammation). Stool samples may be taken per usual protocol, but it is unlikely to aid in the diagnosis. Standard treatment of acute diverticulitis includes the antibiotics metronidazole (Flagyl) and ciprofloxacin (Cipro) along with a restricted diet.

Gastroesophageal reflux disease (GERD)

Essentially, GERD is the flow of contents from the stomach back up into the esophagus. Because the stomach is an acidic environment, GERD often causes a burning type pain in the epigastrium that may radiate up the mid-chest (over the esophagus). Associated symptoms include belching, burping and reflux of stomach acid into the mouth, all of which are highly suggestive of GERD. GERD is often caused by excess secretion of stomach acid after eating, so this pain may be alleviated in the short-term by antacids like TUMS, Zantac or Pepcid. A proton pump inhibitor like omeprazole or Protonix may be taken daily to reduce stomach acid secretion. You will see this on patient medication lists quite frequently.

Peptic Ulcer Disease (PUD)

If a patient experiences chronic GERD or similar acid dysregulation they are at risk for developing an ulcer in the lining of the stomach. Pepsin is a protease (protein-digesting enzyme) found in the stomach and when acid erodes the mucosa of the stomach, pepsin may actually erode the This is a slow process that occurs over a period of weeks or months but may become acute in a matter of days. An ulcer will cause burning pain in the upper abdomen that may briefly subside after eating (as food absorbs much of the stomach acid), but then returns a couple hours later as the stomach empties. The characteristic sign of a peptic ulcer is black, tarry, or coffee-ground like stools called melena. This occurs as the heme molecule in blood (which gives it the red or purple color) is broken down in the intestines and turns black. If left untreated, the patient may lose a significant quantity of blood and become seriously anemic.

Diseases of the Respiratory System

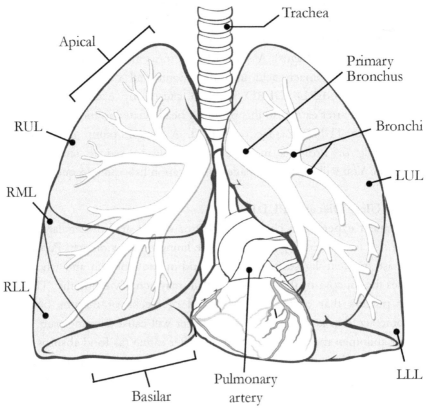

Figure 28: Human lung anatomy. Note there is no left middle lobe (LML) like there is on the right side (RML) but the extra space is used to harbor the heart within the left side of the thorax. Also, note that the terms apical and basilar are often used to refer, respectively, to the top and bottom of the lung fields. This was originally created by Patrick J. Lynch, medical illustrator; C. Carl Jaffe, MD, cardiologist.

Asthma

Asthma is a chronic condition characterized by inflammation, excess mucous secretion and bronchospasm of the small airways of the lungs. This primarily causes dyspnea, wheezing and non-productive coughing. It may be provoked by allergens, irritants, exertion, psychological factors, etc. Physical exam findings may include wheezing, prolonged expiration, and in severe cases use of accessory chest wall muscles to assist with inhalation and exhalation. Patients with intermittent asthma exacerbations may be prescribed a rescue inhaler with the medication albuterol sulfate to be used for acute symptoms. Some patients may need medications to manage their daily asthma symptoms and common medications include Advair and Singulair.

Bronchitis

Bronchitis is the narrowing of the bronchial tree due to inflammation and excess mucus production in the bronchi (the two large air passages after the trachea). The cause of this inflammation may be infectious or allergic. Ninety percent of infectious cases of bronchitis are viral in etiology and are commonly the result of a viral URI that has translocated to the upper part of the lungs. The clinical definition of bronchitis is more simply an intermittently productive cough without evidence of infiltrate (i.e. pneumonia) on a chest x-ray. Additional symptoms may include chest tightness, low-grade fever, and abnormal lung sounds (typically rhonchi) heard during auscultation.

COPD

Chronic obstructive pulmonary disease (COPD) is defined as chronic bronchitis and/or emphysema. These are two separate conditions that each may result from longstanding cigarette use, which can be noted by the number of packs per day (PPD) smoked and number of years, or if multiplied together gives the "pack years" of smoking (e.g. a man that smoked 2 ppd for 35 years has a 70 pack year history of smoking).

Emphysema is a disease characterized by the loss of alveolar elasticity that makes alveoli prone to collapse during exhalation. Collapsed alveoli cannot fill with air and thus do not participate in respiration. However, these alveoli can "pop" back open during inhalation and this popping sound (called crackles) can be heard upon auscultation.

Whereas emphysema involves the lowest portion of the lungs, the alveoli, bronchitis affects the large airways called bronchi. Bronchitis is the inflammation of the bronchi due to an irritant (e.g. allergies, chemicals) or infection. It is defined as a productive cough without evidence of infiltrate on chest x-ray; pneumonia is a productive cough *with* a visual infiltrate on chest x-ray.

There are several different inhaled medications that can be used to treat COPD at home. These can be delivered to the lungs as either a dried powder via an inhaler or as a aerosolized mist by a nebulizer. The most common medications are albuterol, which acts as a short-term rescue inhaler, and Advair, which acts as a long-term maintenance medication.

Obstructive Sleep Apnea

Obstruction of the upper airway while sleeping, generally in apneic (not breathing) periods of 20-40 seconds. Sonorous respirations ("snoring") is indicative of some degree of airway compression that may decompensate into the full blown apneic periods. Often it may be due to an abundance of cervical soft tissue (i.e. neck fat) and requires the use of CPAP while sleeping. CPAP stands for continuous positive airway pressure, which essentially increases the pressure within the airways to help keep them open and prevent these apneic periods. If left untreated, patients may experience excessive daytime fatigue and be at risk for developing atrial fibrillation due to the increased strain of the heart during these apneic episodes. A sleep study is performed by a sleep specialist to confirm this diagnosis and become fitted for CPAP equipment.

Pneumonia

Pneumonia is the inflammation (pneumonitis) of the lungs characterized by consolidation (filling with fluid) of the alveolar air spaces. Because it involves the alveoli, the site of gas exchange, it often causes shortness of breath. It is commonly caused by a viral or bacterial organism and there are two basic types: community acquired pneumonia and hospital-acquired pneumonia. The first is the more simple form and the latter the more complex. Hospital acquired pneumonia is a life-threatening condition often associated with increased antibiotic resistance and virulence. Many people with chronic conditions and thus consistent exposure to health care facilities are at risk for hospital-acquired pneumonia.

Pneumonia may be caused by a combination of factors including impaired protective mechanisms (e.g. poor cough reflex) or immunocompromise as well as exposure to organisms with the means to adhere to and infect the lower respiratory tract. Bacterial pneumonia is often caused by organisms colonizing or originating from the upper airway (nose, mouth and pharynx). This may occur as a result of post-nasal drip common with allergies, upper respiratory infections, and aspiration (accidental inhalation of food particles covered with bacteria from the mouth). Small organisms like bacteria can also hitch a ride on other air particles and navigate through the bronchial tree and lodge themselves in the alveoli. Once there, they may release exotoxins, etc. that cause inflammation to the lung tissue. The inflammatory response recruits immunological cells and also increases vascular permeability, which causes fluid accumulation within the alveoli (consolidation). The thickening of the alveoli (due to inflammation) and presence of fluid (consolidation) impairs gas exchange and causes shortness of breath. In addition, certain toxins or even the organisms themselves may enter the blood stream and cause systemic effects (fever, bacteremia, sepsis).

The diagnosis of pneumonia is part clinical and part radiological. The physical exam can be suggestive of it when crackles are heard on auscultation. The radiological diagnosis is made by the presence of infiltrate on a chest x-ray or CT.

The antibiotic(s) of choice to treat pneumonia differs depending on whether the diagnosis of pneumonia is community or hospital acquired. More simple cases can be treated with oral azithromycin (Zithromax, Z-Pak) or Levaquin, and these are the most frequently encountered antibiotics for pneumonia in the primary care clinic.

Musculoskeletal Conditions

Osteoarthritis (OA) / Degenerative Joint Disease (DJD)

These two conditions are synonymous for a particular type of arthritis. Arthritis can be broken down into "arth" referring to the joints, and "itis" meaning inflammation. Therefore arthritis it "joint inflammation." Osteoarthritis and DJD are more simply known as "wear-and-tear" arthritis. It typically occurs in people as they age and the connective tissue that pads the joints (like the menisci of the knee) wears away. When this occurs, bone-on-bone contact will irritate and inflame the joint and cause pain. Osteoarthritis is often managed with regular use of anti-inflammatories like ibuprofen or Aleve, which are both NSAIDs. There is a risk of kidney damage and GI bleeding with long-term use, something the physician will likely weigh the pros and cons of when discussing the treatment options. Corticosteroid—or simply known as steroid—injections can be given locally to help calm down flares of osteoarthritis. If this pain significantly hampers a patient's quality of life, they made need referral to an orthopedist for further management.

Various conditions: in summary

We cannot explain every single musculoskeletal condition, but below is a list of anatomical structures and the pathology associated with them:

- Bursa and bursitis - bursitis is the inflammation of a bursa, a fluid-filled sac that surrounds a joint and provides padding and lubrication between various joint structures. For example, the pre-patellar bursa is located over the knee cap (a.k.a. the patella) and cushions the bone from pressure applied to the knee cap. It often becomes inflamed from repetitive kneeling and like most cases of bursitis (and inflammation in general), may become swollen, red and painful.

- Ligamentous injuries – this includes minor injuries called sprains and as well as a complete tear of a ligament. The most common ligament injuries occur in these two joints:
  - Knee joint, specifically including the ACL, PCL, LCL, and MCL (anterior, posterior, lateral, medial). Lachman's test may be performed to evaluate for an ACL injury.
  - Ankle joint, specifically including the ligaments adjacent to

the lateral and medial malleoli (malleolus singular, the large bumps on either side of the ankle). These often occur secondary to inversion (foot rolling outward, or severe supination) or eversion (foot rolling inward, or severe pronation) of the ankle.

- Meniscal injuries – the menisci (singular meniscus) are the cartilaginous pads that cushion the knee joint from bone-on-bone contact. There are two per knee (the medial and lateral menisci) and McMurray's test may be performed to help identify a meniscus injury.
- Strains – an injury to a muscle or tendon caused by excess stretching

Diseases of the Urinary Tract

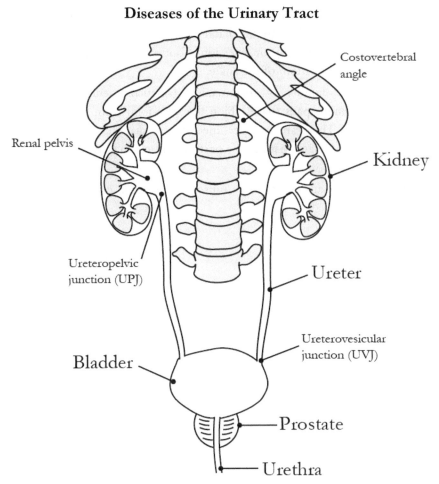

Figure 29: The basic anatomy of the urinary tract: Important landmarks for your purposes include the costovertebral angle (CVA), which is the general location of the kidneys when examining a patient during the physical exam. The CVA may become tender during pyelonephritis—an infection of the renal pelvis ("pyelo" means pelvis). Another important locations are the ureteropelvic junction (UPJ) and ureterovesicular junction (UVJ). These are narrowings in the urinary tract and are common locations for kidney stones to be lodged. Lastly, the prostate is a gland found only in males that surrounds the urethra; it completely surrounds the prostate, but has been uncovered in this diagram.

Benign Prostatic Hyperplasia (BPH)

Also known as an enlarged prostate, BPH is a common non-malignant condition in aging men. Symptoms of an enlarged prostate include slow, weak urine flow as well as urinary urgency and nocturia (needing to wake up at night to urinate).

Urinary Tract Infections

A UTI is caused by the ascension of bacteria through the urinary tract. The source is generally enteric bacteria originating from the bowel or vagina that enter at the distal urethra and ascend to the bladder (cystitis) and even potentially continue up to a kidney (pyelonephritis). UTIs are considerably more frequent in women, as ascending bacteria have a shorter distance to travel in order to reach the bladder. In addition, the prostate gland of men has bactericidal functions.

The inflammation caused by bacterial infection of the urinary tract causes a few well known symptoms, including:

- Dysuria—a burning discomfort during urination
- Urinary frequency—increased frequency of urination
- Urinary urgency—the sensation of needing to urinate often
- Additional symptoms may occur in more severe cases, including hematuria (blood in the urine) and back or flank pain (as in pyelonephritis).

A UTI is defined as a bacterial infection that causes an inflammatory response. Thus, a UTI is defined by the presence of these two items in a urine sample:

- White blood cells
- Bacteria

Pyelonephritis is a more severe UTI in which the infection has spread to the renal pelvis (*"pyelo"* means pelvis). The diagnosis is the same as that of cystitis but patients frequently present with a fever and nearly always have flank pain or CVA tenderness on exam. Antibiotic therapy may differ slightly as well.

If a patient is symptomatic for a UTI and has evidence of WBCs and bacteria in his/her urine, then oral antibiotic therapy is initiated. Common medications that cover the urinary tract include nitrofurantoin (Macrobid), trimethoprim-sulfamethoxazole (Bactrim or Septra), and ciprofloxacin (Cipro). They are generally given for a short course unless the patient has a history of recurrent UTIs. In the case of a more severe UTI (pyelonephritis), IV antibiotics may be required to prevent sepsis.

10. MEDICATIONS

This section will introduce some of the most commonly encountered types of medications in clinic, as well as the particularly common drugs and brand names within each category. Note that the format for naming drugs is to put the generic name first, followed by the capitalized brand name in parenthesis.

The "Must Know" Medications

The medications below will be encountered so frequently that it is essential for the prepared medical scribe to remember the primary use of each. You don't need to understand the dosing or the other minutiae related to each, but if a patient comes into clinic and, for example, Lisinopril is in their medication list, then you should know what condition

1.	Acetaminophen (Tylenol)	an analgesic and antipyretic (fever reducer)
2.	Aspirin	an NSAID that is available as an 81 mg dose (baby aspirin) and 324 mg dose (full aspirin). Unlike other NSAIDs, it is also used to reduce platelet aggregation in cases of a heart attack or stroke
3.	Benadryl	an oral antihistamine that reduces swelling in response to an allergic reaction
4.	Warfarin (Coumadin)	a "blood thinner" taken regularly by patients with a history or risk of forming blood clots (DVT / PE / stroke / afib) to prevent the risk of a future event. The "thinness" of blood is measured every other week with the INR lab test, as too much Coumadin may predispose a person to bleed easily and excessively
5.	Hydrochlorothiazide (HCTZ)	a (thiazide) diuretic used to treat hypertension
6.	Ibuprofen	an NSAID, which acts to reduce pain and inflammation

7. Insulin — the hormone that acts to lower blood sugars and is used to treat hyperglycemia in those with type I and type II diabetes mellitus. There are two major types: fast-acting (taken with meals) and slow-acting (taken in the morning and night)

8. Lasix — a (loop) diuretic used to treat CHF

9. Lisinopril — an ACE (angiotensin-converting enzyme) inhibitor that treats high blood pressure

10. Metformin — the first line medication used to treat type II diabetes, which acts by increasing a person's sensitivity to insulin

11. Metoprolol — the most common beta blocker, a class of medications that reduces blood pressure and slows heart rate most commonly for hypertension and CHF

12. Miralax — a stool softener taken to relieve constipation

13. Nitroglycerin — the sublingual medication used to dilate blood vessels in the case of a heart attack

14. Omeprazole (Prilosec) — a medication that alleviates chronic heartburn by reducing the secretion of gastric acid; it does not immediately relieve symptoms of heartburn (GERD)

15. Ondansetron (Zofran) — the most common medication used to alleviate nausea

16. Prednisone — the most common of the steroids (glucocorticoids), which help to reduce inflammation (e.g. with bronchitis, COPD, etc.)

17. Statins — medications used to treat high cholesterol. There are several brand name statins, but most generic names end in "—statin" (e.g. simvastatin and atorvastatin).

Medication Classes

ACE (Angiotensin-Converting Enzyme) Inhibitors

Block the conversion of angiotensin I to angiotensin II, which is responsible for multiple processes that cause water retention and increased blood pressure. Therefore, ACE inhibitors decrease blood pressure by promoting fluid loss and vasodilation and are used to treat hypertension and CHF. Examples include:

1. Enalapril
2. Lisinopril

Analgesics

Acetaminophen (Tylenol) – an anti-pyretic and pain reliever. It blocks COX-2 activity (see NSAIDs below) in the central nervous system, but given its localized effect is not considered an NSAID.

NSAIDs (Non-Steroidal Anti-Inflammatory Drugs)

Most NSAIDs used in the ED are non-selective, reversible inhibitors of both cyclooxygenase-1 and 2 (COX-1, COX-2) and act as anti-inflammatories and antipyretics. COX-1 is a physiological enzyme with many functions including regulation of gastric acid secretion; its inhibition by NSAIDs is responsible for the common GI side effects of these medications. COX-2 is activated in response to inflammation and has a role in promoting this activity; its inhibition is responsible for the anti-inflammatory effects of NSAIDs. Additional side-effects make NSAIDs unfit for those that are pregnant or have chronic kidney disease.

1. Aspirin – an irreversible COX inhibitor often used as a long-term anticoagulant
2. Ibuprofen (Motrin)
3. Naprosyn (Aleve or Naproxen) – long-acting NSAID taken twice daily; may have greater GI side effects than the shorter acting NSAIDs
4. Ketorolac (Toradol) – an IV NSAID

Narcotics (in order of increasing strength)

These function primarily as analgesics by acting on an opioid receptor in the brain, but they produce multiple side effects due to the activation of opioid receptors in other body regions. By acting at the level of the spinal cord, narcotics may cause respiratory depression. Also, they tend to cause constipation by acting on pre-synaptic neurons in the GI tract. Tolerance and addiction may occur with these medications and they are often prescribed in limited amounts.

1. Tramadol (Ultram) and codeine
2. Hydrocodone-acetaminophen (Vicodin or Norco)
3. Oxycodone-acetaminophen (Percocet)
4. Oxycontin – slow release form
5. Roxicodone (oxycodone) – pure form (no acetaminophen)
6. Hydromorphone (Dilaudid) – quite potent and longer acting than fentanyl; available in oral and IV/IM routes
7. Fentanyl (Sublimaze) – short acting, but very potent

Antithrombotics

Anticoagulants

Prevent the coagulation (clotting) of blood. They are generally used as a prophylactic in those predisposed to forming clots and act by "thinning" the blood and reducing the probability of platelet aggregation (clotting). This includes those with a prior history of blood clots and those with a-fib, CHF, prior strokes or genetic hypercoagulability conditions. This class includes the following medications which all act on different points in the clotting cascade. Common medications in this class are listed below in an order of "increasing strength":

1. Warfarin (Coumadin) – may be counteracted in the case of hemorrhage with fresh frozen plasma and Vitamin K (as its mechanism of action is to impair the activity of Vitamin K).
2. Enoxaparin sodium (Lovenox) – a low-molecular weight heparin administered via intramuscular injection (IM) for short durations before Coumadin reaches effective levels in the blood. It may be only partially counteracted in cases of acute hemorrhage.

Platelet inhibitors

These medications prevent the aggregation of platelets that occurs in response to injury. Unlike anticoagulants, which thin blood as a prophylactic means to reduce the probability of clotting, platelet inhibitors impair the final act of platelet aggregation itself; the extent of impairment is dose dependent. They are often used peri-procedurally when the platelet response is undesirable (such as in the coronary arteries). Because they inhibit platelet aggregation and clotting, any injury sustained while on these medications could have disastrous consequences.

1. Aspirin (ASA) – baby aspirin (81 mg) is often prescribed daily in those with heart disease; full dose (324 mg) is used for acute scenarios

Antihistamines

These block the activity of histamine, a molecule that recruits certain molecules in the body to induce inflammation; this route produces allergic swelling, which is different than traumatic swelling.

H1 blocker

These medications block the histamine-1 (H1) receptor and thus inhibit the activity of histamine.

1. Zantac and Pepcid – these two medications are used commonly to treat heartburn, but are also frequently used in conjunction with H2 blockers to decrease inflammation secondary to histamine release.

H2 blockers

These medications block the histamine-2 (H2) receptor and inhibit the activity of histamine through a separate route than H-1 receptors

1. Diphenhydramine (Benadryl)
2. Loratadine (Claritin) – a long-acting antihistamine
3. Cetirizine (Zyrtec) – a long-acting antihistamine

Beta-blockers

Block the activity of epinephrine—a vasoconstrictor—by binding to the beta-adrenergic receptor that binds to epinephrine. Because these receptors exist in various locations throughout the body, certain beta-blockers may have greater activity on specific organs or systems. In general, the most common therapeutic uses include:

1. Hypertension – promotes vasodilation and therefore decrease blood pressure. In this same manner, they may be used for migraine prophylaxis by causing vasodilation of cerebral arteries.

2. CHF – slows electrical conduction at the sinus node and AV node, allowing for greater filling during diastole and an increased ejection fraction. It may be used in combination with standard ACE inhibitor and diuretic therapies.

3. Arrhythmias – slows electrical conduction in the sinus node and AV node, reducing heart rate and restoring a more regular rhythm in various tachyarrhythmias.

Specific drugs include:
1. Atenolol
2. Carvedilol (Coreg)
3. Metoprolol

Calcium-Channel Blockers (CCBs)

These medications block the activity of voltage-dependent calcium channels, which are present in cardiac muscle cells as well as the smooth muscle of blood vessels. By reducing the activity of these, Ca^{2+} channel blockers reduce heart rate by reducing voltage conduction from the SA and AV nodes to the ventricles and are used to treat tachyarrhythmias. By the same mechanism, CCBs cause arterial vasodilation and may be used to counteract high blood pressure and angina pectoris. Different classes of CCBs are more specific for cardiac tissue or acting peripherally. Examples include:

1. Amlodipine (Norvasc) – a long-acting CCB
2. Diltiazem (Cardizem)

Contraception

Oral contraceptive pills (OCPs) are a very common method of birth control. OCPs contain estrogens, progesterones or both. Often times the names will have numbers and slashes indicating the relative doses of steroids. Below we have listed some common OCPs.

- Ortho Novum 1/35
- Ortho Tri-cyclen
- Loestrin 1/20
- Yasmin

In addition to OCPs there are other forms of birth control including:

- Depo Provera – injection of a progesterone every three months
- Norplant – subcutaneous implant that lasts 5 years
- Nuva Ring – a ring inserted into the vagina once a month and releases hormones
- Mirena – a hormone-releasing intrauterine device (IUD)
- Paraguard – an IUD that does not release hormones

Diuretics

Medications that induce diuresis, or urine production, to reduce the volume of bodily fluids in those with hypertension, congestive heart failure (CHF), chronic kidney disease (CKD) or other renal or cardiovascular conditions.

1. Hydrochlorothiazide (HCTZ) – a thiazide diuretic
2. Lasix – a loop diuretic

Functional Medication Classes

Antacids

This group of medications mitigate the symptoms of indigestion, heartburn, and acid reflux (GERD). They include over the counter medications taken as necessary or prescribed medications for chronic problems.

1. Tums – made of calcium carbonate ($CaCO_3$), these are taken during symptoms of heartburn as carbonate is a base that in the presence of acid (H^+), forms the buffer bicarbonate (HCO_3^-)
2. Omeprazole (Prilosec) – a proton-pump inhibitor (PPI), it reduces the secretion of acid from the parietal cells of the stomach and are taken on a regular basis rather than when symptoms occur

Antiemetics

Medications used to counteract nausea and vomiting (emesis). The medications below represent a functional category but do not act on similar physiological processes.

1. Meclizine (Antivert) – the original anti-vertigo medicine that is available as a generic medication
2. Ondansetron (Zofran) – a newer anti-emetic that is available in oral, sublingual, or IV forms
3. Promethazine (Phenergan) – an anti-histamine (H1 blocker) used as an antiemetic; other antihistamines may be used for this same reason

Laxatives, Stool Softeners and Suppositories

These medications promote the passage and output of stool. There are two common types of laxatives, as detailed below:

1. Stool softeners – compounds that are taken orally and are insoluble in the human GI tract. They cause the retention of fluid within the GI tract and thus soften stool for easier passage. They may be taken daily for the treatment of chronic constipation and usually produce a BM in 1-3 days.
   a. Prune juice
   b. Miralax (most common type)
   c. Docusate (Colace)
2. Osmotic laxatives – compounds that act as stool softeners (as they too are poorly absorbed in the gut) but also stimulate the release of water and electrolytes into the intestinal tract. They act quicker than stool softeners (< 6 hours), but may also cause some discomfort and cramping.
   a. Milk of magnesia (MOM)
   b. Magnesium citrate
3. Stimulant laxatives – compounds that increase the contractility of the intestines. This type acts more quickly that osmotic laxatives but are not indicated in those with obstruction or impaction.
   a. Bisacodyl (Dulcolax)
   b. Senokot
4. Suppositories – technically, this refers to any medication given rectally. Enemas are suppositories meant to hydrate stool in the distal rectum and promote defecation. Common types include mineral oil, saline, glycerol and barium.

Glucocorticoids (steroids)

Anti-inflammatory molecules / medications used to treat a wide variety of conditions. In addition, they tend to increase blood glucose levels, which may be apparent in diabetic patients taking glucocorticoids. Common forms, in an order of increasing strength, are listed below:

1. Cortisol – the human body's natural glucocorticoid
2. Prednisone – converted to prednisolone in the liver

3. Prenisolone – the active metabolite of prednisone
4. Methylprednisolone (Solu-Medrol)
5. Dexamethasone – a potent anti-inflammatory, several times stronger than methylprednisolone

Glucose Regulation

For patients with type I or type II diabetes mellitus, there are several classes of medications available as well as fast-acting and slow-acting insulin products. In general, these are the most common medications and medication types:

1. Metformin – first line treatment for diabetes, decreases glucose production by the liver
2. Basal insulin products – these are slow-acting forms of insulin that provide a baseline level of insulin throughout the day
   a. Lantus
3. Prandial insulin products – these are fast-acting and are taken at meal-time to counteract short-term blood sugar spikes
   a. Novolog
   b. Humalog

Nitrates

These medications produce nitric oxide, an endogenous vasodilator (through debatable mechanisms), and are therefore used in the treatment of hypertension, angina and acute myocardial infarctions. Common examples include:

1. Isosorbide mononitrate (Imdur) – indicated for prophylaxis of angina
2. Nitroglycerin – primarily use is as a short-acting vasodilator, as consistent use over 2-3 weeks may induce tolerance.

Selective Serotonin Reuptake Inhibitors (SSRIs)Error! Bookmark not defined.

SSRIs increase the amount of serotonin circulating between neurons in the brain. They are most commonly used to treat depression, more technically called major depressive disorder or major depression, but are also frequently used for anxiety disorders as well. The most common drugs include:

1. Citalopram (Celexa)

2. Escitalopram (Lexapro)
3. Fluoxetine (Prozac)
4. Paroxetine (Paxil)
5. Sertraline (Zoloft)
6. Venlafaxine (Effexor)

Statins

Limit the endogenous production of cholesterol by inhibiting the key enzyme (HMG-CoA reductase) and hence act to reduce cholesterol in those with hypercholesteremia. Common examples include:

1. Atorvastatin (Lipitor)
2. Rosuvastatin (Crestor)
3. Simvastatin (Zocor)

Topical Creams

There are several topical (on the skin) medications that can be used for various types of rashes. The most common medications and their uses are as follows:

1. Hydrocortisone – a steroid medication (note cortisone is similar to cortisol, the body's natural steroid). It is typically used for rashes that are non-infectious in origin, like a reactive dermatitis (e.g. poison ivy) or eczema.
2. Barrier creams (e.g. Desitin, Vaseline) – these are commonly used to prevent physical irritation of the skin. In infants, they may be used to treat diaper rash.
3. Antifungals (e.g. Lotrimin) – treat fungal infections of the skin, which normally are scaly in appearance and may seem similar to eczema. Fungal infections may be diagnosed by scraping cells onto a microscope slide and adding KOH (potassium hydroxide), which degrades skin and hair but leaves fungi intact and can therefore be seen under a microscope.

There are many more medications that you will come across in your time as a scribe. Luckily, much of your time as a scribe will be spent on the computer and thus you have the ability to look-up other medications on an as needed basis.

Vaccines/Immunizations

Immunizations are highly effective at limited infectious disease and even cervical cancer in the case of HPV vaccines. As a scribe you should be at least familiar with both the names and abbreviations of the common immunizations listed here:

1. Hepatitis B (HBV)
2. Diphtheria-tetanus-acellular pertussis (DTaP)
3. Hemophilus influenza type B (Hib)
4. Inactivated polio vaccine (IPV)
5. Measles-mumps-rubella (MMR)
6. Varicella-zoster virus (VZV)
7. Pneumococcal conjugate vaccine (PCV)
8. Hepatitis A (HAV)
9. Influenza
10. Rotavirus
11. Meningococcal polysaccharide vaccine (MPSV4)
12. Human papilloma virus (HPV)

Antibiotics

Antibiotics effect different organisms depending on the nature of the organism (aerobic, anaerobic, gram positive, gram negative). When taken orally, certain antibiotics are taken up into the body and others remain within the GI tract (like vancomycin, hence why it is used to treat C.diff colitis). Once an antibiotic is in the systemic circulation it may localize to a particular tissue, and thus certain antibiotics are prescribed for infections of particular tissues (e.g. azithromycin for bronchitis as it "covers" the respiratory tract). Antibiotics are generally thought of as being "stronger" when they cover a wide range of organisms (a.k.a. broad spectrum) and have lower rates of antimicrobial resistance. The table on the next page gives an overview of some of the most typical uses for common antibiotics.

CLASS	DRUG	COMMON INDICATIONS
CARBAPENEMS	Imipenem-cilastatin (Primaxin)	Lungs, skin, intra-abdominal infections, gynecologic infections, UTI
CEPHALOSPORINS: 1st Generation	cephalexin (Keflex)	Cellulitis, abscesses of the skin
	cefazolin (Ancef)	
2nd Generation	cefprozil (Cefzil)	Respiratory infections, skin, otitis media, pharyngitis / tonsillitis
3rd Generation	cefdinir (Omnicef)	Community-acquired pneumonia, sinusitis, skin
	ceftriaxone (Rocephin)	
GLYCOPEPTIDES	vancomycin (Vancocin)	C.diff colitis (oral only), cellulitis, second line for pneumonia
LINCOSAMIDES	Clindamycin (Cleocin)	cellulitis, second line for penicillin allergies
MACROLIDES	azithromycin (Zithromax)	Upper-and lower-respiratory tract infections
NITROFURANS	nitrofurantoin (Macrobid)	Cystitis
NITROIMIDAZOLE	metronidazole (Flagyl)	C.diff colitis, bacterial vaginosis
QUINOLONES	ciprofloxacin (Cipro)	UTI, community acquired pneumonia, bacterial diarrhea
	levofloxacin (Levaquin)	
PENICILLINS	Amoxicillin	Ear infections, sinus infections, wide range generally
	amoxicillin-clavulanate (Augmentin)	
	ampicillin-sulbactam (Unasyn)	ABX resistant organisms
	piperacillin-tazobactam (Zosyn)	Pyelonephritis, hospital acquired pneumonia
SULFONAMIDES	trimethoprim-sulfamethoxazole (Bactrim)	UTI, COPD/bronchitis, MRSA cellulitis
TETRACYLCINES	doxycycline (Vibramycin)	Bronchitis/COPD,

11. LABORATORY RESULTS

Below is a brief overview of the most common, meaningful labs for the young scribe. Some labs are ordered in a package such as the "complete blood count" also known as the CBC. Other labs are ordered individually. We have tried to go through all the most common labs ordered in the primary care clinic.

It should be noted that different settings may use slightly different lab technology to perform these tests and the normal range as well as the units may vary.

Pathology	Corresponding Lab Marker
Anticoagulation (Coumadin monitoring)	INR
Blood clots (pulmonary embolism and DVT)	D-dimer
Blood sugar (average)	Hemoglobin A1C (HbA1C)
Congestive heart failure (fluid overload)	BNP (brain natriuretic peptide)
Infection (general)	WBCs (leukocytes)
Inflammation (systemic)	CRP (C-reactive protein) ESR (erythrocyte sedimentation rate)
Kidney function	Creatinine GFR BUN
Myocardial infarction	Troponin
Pancreatic function	Lipase
Septic shock	Lactate
Urinary tract infection	Bacteria and WBCs (in UA)

The CBC, or complete blood count, is ordered for many reasons on a wide array of patients. It has four major components: white blood count (WBC), hemoglobin (HGB), hematocrit (HCT) and platelets (PLT). It may also be ordered with a "differential" that further breaks down the white blood count into separate types of white blood cells, collectively known as leukocytes.

Hemoglobin and Red Blood Cells

Hemoglobin is the functional unit of red blood cells and decreased hemoglobin impairs the ability of red blood cells to carry oxygen.

Anemia

Low hemoglobin is traditionally called anemia but more generally it may be defined as either low hemoglobin or low RBCs. A normal range for hemoglobin, depending on your age and sex is 12-17g/dL. However, it is really only important to note when significantly below normal values; a rule of thumb is that Hgb < 10.0 is significant.

A few of the many subtypes of anemia include:

- Acute blood loss anemia: low hemoglobin and RBCs due to excessive blood loss and/or dilution. Common causes are trauma, internal bleeding, menstruation and IV fluid rehydration.
- Chronic blood loss via heavy menses (menstrual periods).
- Hemolytic anemia: breakdown of RBCs, commonly due to an infectious agent (e.g. malaria)
- Iron-deficient anemia: Lack of dietary iron prevents production of hemoglobin
- Pernicious anemia: Lack of vitamin B12 absorption due to a lack of intrinsic factor secreted from parietal cells of the gastric mucosa. This may be result from an autoimmune condition (i.e. Crohn's) or following gastric bypass surgery.

Platelets (PLT)

Thrombocytopenia

Decreased levels of blood platelets as a result of impaired production or increased hemolysis (breakdown). Causes may include autoimmune problems, genetic disorders, leukemia, lupus, chemotherapeutics or dietary inadequacies.

Thrombocythemia (a.k.a. thrombocytosis)
Elevated levels of blood platelets that increases the tendency of blood to form clots.

White Blood Cells
The group of cells responsible for the immune response and defending the body from infection.

Leukopenia
Depressed levels of WBCs, a marker of immunocompromise or some viral infections.

Leukocytosis
Elevated white count due to infection or stress, generally (virus, bacteria, fungi, other).

CBC with differential or "the diff" is the breakdown into what types of WBCs are present in a given sample. It is usually divided into percentages and then an "absolute count," the actual number of a given cell type in a certain volume. There are a few important types of white blood cells: neutrophils, lymphocytes, eosinophils and monocytes. The differential may also further break these WBCs down into different developmental subtypes such as "bands" (immature), myelocytes, etc.

Neutrophils
Neutrophils are the primary white blood cells produced in response to bacterial reactions or acute inflammation (e.g. MI).

Neutrophilia
Elevated relative amount of neutrophils in the blood (> 72%). A "Left shift" is a subcategorization marked by an increased percentage of immature neutrophils in the blood, possibly reflecting a bone marrow disorder.

Neutropenia
Abnormally low-levels of neutrophils (a type of WBC), which makes one

susceptible to bacterial infections. There are three stages of classification based on the absolute neutrophil count (ANC) per microliter of blood, which corresponds to the associated risk of infection:

Basic metabolic panel (BMP) (also called the chem 7, chem 8, or other names) is a set of tests that essentially measures a patient's electrolytes. There are several components to most "panels."

Sodium (Na)
Hypernatremia
High sodium levels (above 145 mEq/L) may be seen in dehydration or endocrine abnormalities.

Hyponatremia
Low sodium levels (below 135 mEq/L) may be seen in psychogenic polydipsia (drinking way too much water) and other endocrine abnormalities. It can lead to seizures and altered mental status when severe.

Potassium (K)
Hypokalemia
Low circulating potassium levels (< 3.5 mEq/L). Potassium is a requirement for maintenance of membrane potentials and molecular transport; low-levels may cause increasingly severe symptoms ranging from fatigue, to arrhythmias and respiratory depression as various muscles cells in the body experience dysfunction. It is frequently caused by induced-diuresis or poor intake.

Hyperkalemia
High circulating potassium levels (> 5.0 mEq/L). Elevated potassium levels disrupt the membrane potential across skeletal and cardiac muscle cells (secondary to increased extracellular potassium) and cause the most notable symptoms in these systems. Mild hyperkalemia may cause malaise, palpitations, and arrhythmias; severe hyperkalemia (>6.5 mEq/L) may result in ventricular fibrillation or asystole.

Creatinine (Cr)
Creatinine is a normal product of muscle breakdown. Blood creatinine level

is generally considered a measure of kidney function. A creatinine of 1.0 is normal; this has been standardized in most labs so that this is the case.

Renal dysfunction
An elevated creatinine indicates renal function is lower than normal as the kidneys are less able to clear creatinine from the body.

Low creatinine
A low creatinine indicates the patient has little muscle; otherwise it is not diagnostically significant for most patients

BUN

BUN (blood urea nitrogen) is another indicator of renal function. Urea, like creatinine, is consistently being filtered by the kidneys. However, whereas creatinine has a fixed rate of reabsorption in the nephron (unit of the kidney) and is filtered from the blood at a constant rate, urea reabsorption is constantly regulated.

Dehydration
When blood water volume is low as in dehydration, the concentration of BUN reaching the kidneys is increased. This causes increased reabsorption of urea in the nephron; in contrast creatinine absorption is relatively stable. Thus, an elevated "BUN/creatinine ratio" can be a good indicator of dehydration, defined as BUN : Creatinine > 20.

Renal dysfunction
If the creatinine is elevated and the BUN : Creatinine ratio is low (< 10), then renal dysfunction is present. This suggests that urea is being minimally reabsorbed in the nephron as a result of renal dysfunction. This is helpful to differentiate between an elevated creatinine due to dehydration and that due to primary renal dysfunction.

Other Labs

(Cardiac) Troponin

Troponin is one of the molecules fundamental to skeletal and cardiac muscle contraction via the actin-myosin mechanism.

Myocardial infarction

As it is found in muscle tissue, the presence of elevated troponin levels in the blood is diagnostically useful for identifying breakdown of muscle; the troponin I and troponin T subtypes are specific for identifying myocardial breakdown and are a common indicator of myocardial cell death seen during heart attacks

D-dimer

Blood clots are made up of an interconnected network of the protein fibrin. When enzymes degrade this clot matrix, it breaks the clot into fragments containing two "D" fragments of the fibrin molecule.

DVT/PE

Because the d-dimer is a measure of clot breakdown, a high d-dimer represents an active clotting process such as venous thromboembolism, pulmonary embolism, or may even be positive from an extensive bruise.

Glucose

Blood or serum glucose is simply the amount of sugar present in the blood stream. It is generally only abnormal in those with diabetes type I or type II. Normal fasting (no recent food) glucose is 70-100, but frequently blood is drawn for testing when patients are not fasting so mildly elevated values are not concerning.

Hyperglycemia

If insulin production is inadequate (type I) or the body's sensitivity to insulin is poor, then hyperglycemia ensues. This may be exacerbated by the use of steroids (glucocorticoids) or active infection. There exists a spectrum of severity, but hyperglycemia is defined as > 200 mg/dl, though symptoms may not appear until even higher.

Hypoglycemia

Accidental overuse of synthetic insulins may cause hypoglycemia (Glu < 60).

Hemoglobin A1C

Also known as glycosylated hemoglobin, this lab reflects the average blood glucose over the past 3 months and is useful for diabetic monitoring, since a single blood glucose reading may fluctuate through a wide range for the individual.

INR (International Normalized Ratio)

Measures the extrinsic clotting pathway (factors I, II, V, VII, X), which is affected by Coumadin use, liver damage and Vitamin K deficiencies.

Supratherapeutic INR

Elevated levels (> 1.3) represent greater clotting time ("thinned blood"). In patients with atrial fibrillation, the ideal range is 2.0 – 2.5 to reduce the risk of thrombosis and a supratherapeutic INR is considered > 2.5.

Subtherapeutic INR

Low levels (< 0.9) represent increased susceptibility to thrombosis ("thickened blood")

12. BILLING AND CODING

Primary Care Billing and Coding

As a scribe in the primary care setting it is important that you have an understanding of billing and coding. Billing is the mechanism by which third parties (patients, private insurance, medicare/medicaid) are charged for services. Coding is assigning of specific codes to a patient visit to designate what type of services were provided in the clinic.

ICD-10 is the tenth version of the International Classification of Disease, created by the WHO. This is replacing ICD-9 and is much more complex. Essentially, these numeric codes are assigned to any diagnosis/condition that the patient has—past or present. These codes are used to justify billing of a CPT code(s) to the third-party payers.

Current procedural terminology (CPT) codes are very important from a billing standpoint. These are 5-digit codes for procedures and services provided by the care provider, clinic or hospital. All CPT codes must be justified by appropriate ICD-10 diagnoses or symptoms. This is called medical necessity and is required for payment.

Important CPT codes include evaluation and management codes (E/M codes). These codes are a basic charge applied for most patients based on the complexity of the patient evaluation and whether or not the patient is new or established. Generally each patient evaluated in the primary care clinic will be assigned an E/M code, in addition to any other procedure CPT codes based on procedures performed during the visit.

As an example, a 75 year old male comes into clinic with knee pain and swelling. While in the clinic the physician performs a knee aspiration and the patient also receives a Pneumovax vaccination as he was overdue for the pneumococcal vaccine. Three different CPT codes would apply to this patient, including:
1) an E/M code for the general evaluation of the patient
2) a CPT code for the knee needle aspiration and
3) a medication code for the vaccine.

It is important that you as a scribe understand how this works so that your documentation reflects the appropriate services. In this case the E/M level will be determined by the complete nature of the note generated by the scribe. The CPT code for the knee aspiration will be dependent on the procedure note documented by the scribe and the medication code cannot be assigned unless it is documented in the patient's note by the scribe. As you can see the scribe's attention to detail is vital for coding and billing in the primary care clinic.

The E/M Codes

A more in depth understanding of the evaluation and management (E/M) codes is important for scribes. These codes are also sometimes called "the level of service." There are three important items to determine the appropriate E/M level of care.

- Is this an inpatient or outpatient visit?
- Is it a new or established patient?
- How complex is the evaluation of the patient?

Below is a chart of the E/M codes most likely used in the primary care clinic setting. Obviously, in the clinic setting a scribe will be dealing exclusively with patients on an outpatient basis; that is, they are not admitted to the hospital (inpatient), but we have included the E/M codes for the hospital here to be complete.

E/M Codes:

Level	Outpatient New	Outpatient Established	Inpatient New	Inpatient Established
1	99201	99211	99221	99231
2	99202	99212	99222	99232
3	99203	99213	99223	99233
4	99204	99214		
5	99205	99215		

A new patient is defined as a patient that has not been seen by anyone in the billing physician's practice group in the last 3 years. So hypothetically a patient already seen by the provider could be characterized as a "new" patient. New patient E/M codes bill at a higher level than established patients, which is understandable because the physician must take more time to acquaint themselves with a new patient than with an established patient. Within patient groups (new or established), the higher the complexity of the patient, the higher the E/M level and the more the provider is able to bill for the services.

The overall complexity of the patient for determining the appropriate E/M level is determined by:

- Patient history components
- Physical exam components
- Medical decision making (MDM) complexity

The billing criteria for the five billing levels is mildly different for new patient visits and established patient visits. In general, new patient visits require more information for any given billing level. Below is a table of the component requirements to bill at a given E/M level for new patient visits. All of the criteria for a given level must be met to permit the assignment of that code for the patient's visit. Note that for the physical exam there must be two documented findings (e.g. soft, non-tender) within a given physical exam system (e.g. the gastrointestinal system).

New Patient Billing Criteria:

	Level 1 99201	Level 2 99202	Level 3 99203	Level 4 99204	Level 5 99205
CC	+	+	+	+	+
History:					
HPI	1	1	4	4	4
ROS	0	1	2	10	10
PMH/FH /SH	0	0	1	3	3
Physical Exam	1 system	2 systems	6 systems	9 systems	9 systems
MDM Complexity	Minimal	Minimal	Low	Moderate	Complex

Established Patient Billing Criteria:

	Level 1 99211	Level 2 99212	Level 3 99214	Level 4 99214	Level 5 99215
CC	+	+	+	+	+
History:					
HPI	NA	1	1	4	4
ROS	NA	0	1	2	10
PMH/FH /SH	NA	0	0	1	2
Physical Exam	NA	1 system	6 systems	6 systems	9 systems
MDM Complexity	NA	Minimal	Low	Moderate	Complex

E/M level 1 is of minimal importance and mainly pertains to isolated nursing visits. A focus on levels 2-5 is prudent.

Next, we will discuss the above chart from top to bottom. The chief complaint (**CC**) is absolutely required on all patient visits, whether new or established. Most EMRs require this field, but as a scribe you should be certain that all patients have a chief complaint. A chief complaint of simply "follow-up" is not adequate and must be further explained. "Follow-up, hypertension" is acceptable.

The history components include the history of present illness (HPI), review of systems and the group called PMH/FH/SH—the past medical history, family history and social history.

HPI components include description of the patient's pain or symptoms. This includes the OPQRSTA qualifiers—time of onset, palliative or provocative factors, quality of the pain, region or location of the pain, severity of the pain, timing, and associated symptoms. Review the HPI section of the book if you do not recall these characteristics of the HPI. So for example, the brief HPI that follows contains 4 HPI components:

A 17 year-old male presents with sharp, severe left ankle pain after twisting his ankle one hour ago. He also complains of numbness in the foot. The pain is much worse with walking and weight bearing.

This patient would meet HPI criteria for a level 4 or 5 visit assuming all of the other criteria are met.

Some more chronic conditions are not amenable to the above descriptors so it is acceptable in this case to state whether they are improved, stable or worsening. Documentation of 3 or more chronic conditions and the current status of the conditions can replace a 4-component HPI from a billing standpoint.

The review of systems (**ROS**) is also important for billing levels 3-5. There are 14 systems that are recognized by CMS for the review of systems as noted below:

- Constitutional
- Eyes
- ENT
- Cardiovascular
- Respiratory
- Gastrointestinal (GI)
- Genitourinary (GU)
- Musculoskeletal
- Neurologic
- Integumentary/Breast
- Psychiatric
- Hematologic/Lymphatic
- Endocrine
- Immunologic/Allergic

You can see on the table on the previous page the number of ROS components that must be included for a given E/M level. A "catch-all" phrase such as "a complete ROS was obtained and negative" is sometimes used in lieu of a complete 14 system ROS. It should also be noted that ROS requirements can be completed using a patient filled-out form as long as it is documented in the chart that "the complete ROS form completed by the patient was reviewed by the physician."

In the same table above you will notice that the **PMH/FH/SH** components are only pertinent for E/M levels 4 and 5. Each of the PMH, FH, and SH count as their own component. Only one of these three items is required for an E/M level 4 and 2 for the level 5 code.

For the **physical exam**, like the ROS, there are CMS-recognized systems that count towards billing and as many as nine of these are necessary to meet level 5 billing requirements. The 12 CMS-recognized physical exam sections include:

- Constitutional/Vitals
- Eyes
- ENT
- Cardiovascular
- Respiratory
- Gastrointestinal
- Genitourinary
- Musculoskeletal
- Integumentary (Skin) or Breast
- Neurologic
- Psychiatric
- Hematologic/Lymphatic

As you can see in our favorite table, the number listed represents the total number of physical exam elements that must be present for a given level. For E/M level 4, at least 12 total exam elements are required across two or more systems. For the level 5 chart at least 2 elements are required in each of 9 or more systems (a minimum of 18 total elements).

Lastly, the **medical decision making or MDM**, has three components that are used in the billing process including the:

- Number of diagnoses/problems
- Review of data
- Risk

For each diagnosis it is important to document if the condition is 1) new or established and 2) stable, deteriorated, or improved. As a scribe, it is important that you capture all diagnoses from the conversation between the physician and patient and attach appropriate qualifiers (e.g. chronic hypertension, worsening) to appropriately code for a patient visit. Using these details, a "coder" will use an algorithmic point system to determine the patient's complexity. A total of 4 or more points from the list below qualifies as a complex MDM and therefore meets higher billing requirements.

- Minor problem= 1 point
- Establish problem (stable or improving)= 1 point
- Establish problem (worsening)= 2 points
- New problem without planned evaluation= 3 points
- New problem with plan= 4 point

Data reviewed is another important component to determine the complexity of the MDM. Examples of this include the review of radiology tests, labs, EKGs, or even a review of outside medical records (from another hospital or clinic). As a scribe, it is important to recognize that adding a little phrase about the review of current tests and/or outside records may impact the billing level for that patient. Some EMRs are quite good at integrating these occurrences in the note, whereas other will require you to do so manually. A point system is also used in data review with one pain equating to minimal complexity for MDM, two point is low complexity, 3 points is moderate and 4 point is equivalent to complex MDM (see the original master chart for the MDM requirements for a given E/M level). Below is how the points are assigned for data review:

- Radiology tests (US, x-rays, CT, MRI)= 1 point
- Lab test reviewed= 1point
- Independent review of X-ray or EKG= 2 points
- Review of test with other physician that performed the test= 1 point
- Attempt to obtain outside records= 1 point
- Review/summary of outside records= 1 point

Risk is the final component considered in the complexity of the MDM.

Generally speaking the risk can be based on the severity of the problem, such as immediate suicidal thoughts (very high risk); invasiveness of tests, such as coronary angiography (high risk); or the risks of a given treatment. Higher risk treatments include medications that require extensive monitoring, such as warfarin or other anticoagulant therapy. It is important as a scribe that you cue in on any risk-based discussion or dictation by the provider. If any component is high risk, the entire visit is deemed high risk.

In order for a chart to meet the MDM requirements for an E/M level 5, the patient must meet the criteria in at least 2 of the 3 MDM categories:

- Complexity of the problem as determined by points
- Complexity of the data reviewed as determined by points
- A high risk problem, procedure or treatment

In addition to basic E/M codes, counseling is also sometimes added as a CPT code. In order to bill for counseling at least 50% of the patient encounter must be face-to-face counseling directly between the patient and the physician. The total time spent counseling the patient must also be documented and this is typically inserted quite explicitly at the bottom of the note.

As a scribe it is not necessary to memorize every detail of billing and coding, but if you choose to master this material it will serve you well as a scribe and into your career as a medical professional since these medical economics items are generally quite neglected in medical education programs.

APPENDIX A: SAMPLE HPI LIBRARY

In this section we have compiled several more example H&Ps, progress notes, and discharge summaries to help further familiarize you with the level of detail within each. Note the differences between each type of note as you read

ER Notes: Chest Pain

The first two examples in this section will cover the most important features of a chest pain HPI to rule out a myocardial infarction and pulmonary embolism. The first one below is an HPI for a patient with chest pain who is actually having a myocardial infarction (MI, "heart attack). This is the classic story for a patient having an MI with important historical features that should be included in the chest pain patient's HPI if they are elicited by the physician.

> John Smithson is a 55 year-old male smoker, with a history of hypertension and diabetes, who presents with gradual onset of severe, ongoing left sub-sternal chest pressure associated with diaphoresis and shortness of breath The pressure started while he was walking up stairs approximately 30 minutes prior to arrival in the ED. It is greatest at the left sternal border and seems to radiate into the left arm and neck. The pain has subsided to 5/10 in severity since, though nothing seemed to make it obviously better or worse. Patient denies similar pain in the past. Patient has no known previous cardiac events or workup. There is no family history of early cardiac disease. No h/o hyperlipidemia.

Note that this accurately captured the pertinent negatives, which are often the most easily forgotten details. The last few sentences address these pertinent negatives in regard to:
- prior chest pain
- previous cardiac workups (EKGs, echocardiograms, stress tests, etc.)
- And the remaining risk factors for CAD (family history, hyperlipidemia)

All chest pain patients should have their possible risk factors for cardiac disease included in their HPI. Risk factors are cigarette smoking, hypertension, diabetes, hypercholesteremia/ hyperlipidemia and family history of premature coronary artery disease in parents or siblings (i.e. <55 years in first degree male or <65 years in females). Hormone replacement therapy is also a risk factor for women, as is being post-menopausal.

Here is an HPI from another patient with chest pain who is suffering from a pulmonary embolism and associated deep vein thrombosis (DVT).

This 60 yo female presents with sudden onset of sharp, left lateral chest pain associated with significant SOB and dizziness beginning 30 minutes PTA. Pain is non-radiating pleuritic. Patient has never had this type of pain before. She relates that she was on a 12 hour plane trip to the Far East last week and developed a large amount of swelling and pain in her right calf 3 days ago. She is a smoker with no h/o HTN, hypercholesterolemia or diabetes. No family h/o early CAD or coagulopathies.

With the following X HPIs try and determine the most likely cause of the patient's symptoms. Note that most will follow the traditional chronological order of writing the HPI and will expose you to the general flow and terminology that is acceptable. Good luck!

HPI #1: John Doe is a 57 year old male, with a history of hypertension, diabetes type I and smoking, who presents with left sided exertional chest pain. He was running on a treadmill this morning at 0800 (3 hours PTA) when the pressure-like pain began with associated symptoms of nausea and light-headedness. Pain resolved after 5 minutes of resting and recurred while walking up the stairs while exiting the gym. Since that time the pain has diminished and he is currently pain free. No history of similar pain in the past. He takes metoprolol for hypertension and smokes 1 ppd. No h/o hyperlipidemia or family h/o heart disease.

HPI #2: John Doe is a 52 yo male smoker with a history of hypertension who presents after sudden onset of severe, crushing, chest pain that woke him from sleep this morning. Pain was located at the left sternal border and radiated into the left arm. At onset, he took 81 mg ASA and called 911 for EMS transport to the ED. EMS noted the pt to be diaphoretic, gave him 1 x NTG and pain slightly improved in route. Currently he complains of difficulty catching his breath and nausea. No history of similar pain in the past. No family h/o of an early life cardiac event.

HPI #3: Jane Doe is a 21 yo female who presents with gradually worsening central chest pain over the last few days. Pain is sharp in nature and worse with deep breathing. She notes it is slightly tender as well. No cough, fever or chills. H/o similar pain in the past, lasted a few days, then went away.

HPI #4: Juan Doe is a 17 yo male who presents with sudden onset of severe right sided chest pain and shortness of breath. He was performing full contact drills at football practice this afternoon and was hit by another player in the right chest when symptoms began. He complains of chest pain that is sharp and pleuritic. No history of similar pain.

HPI #5: John Doe is a 39 yo male, s/p uneventful left TKA 1 week ago who presents with severe right-sided chest pain that radiates into his back. The pain began suddenly approximately one hour ago while at rest and is rated 10/10 in severity, worsened with deep breathing. He complains of SOB and tachycardia and notes an area of tenderness and swelling in the right calf that began 3 days ago. No hemoptysis. No h/o similar pain. No h/o coagulopathy. The patient actively smokes and reportedly has a family history of blood clot problems.

Chest pain Answers

1. ***Stable angina.*** *You have read and seen plenty about stable angina as a sign of coronary artery disease, so hopefully this was an easy one for you. You may have thought this was considered an acute MI, but stable angina occurs due to relative ischemia in a coronary artery whereas an acute MI is caused by the total occlusion and ischemia of a coronary artery.*

2. ***Acute myocardial infarction (AMI).*** *This should be fairly straightforward. Many of his symptoms are classical for an acute MI, including diaphoresis, nausea, and pain that subsides after taking aspiring and/or nitroglycerin.*

3. ***Costochondritis***

4. ***Traumatic pneumothorax.*** *This is a subtype of pneumothorax in which a person with healthy lungs suffers a rib fracture due to trauma, which then likely punctured part of the right lung and led to the pneumothorax.*

5. ***Pulmonary embolism (PE).*** *This patient has several risk factors for a PE including a habit of smoking, a positive family history, and recent surgery. He may not have the tell-tale sign of hemoptysis, but remember this is not always present; it is a very specific sign, but low sensitivity.*

ER Notes: Respiratory Complaints

HPI #1: Joseph M Doe is a 15 year old male with a h/o asthma who presents with wheezing, chest tightness, and shortness of breath beginning last night. There was no discernible trigger precipitating onset of symptoms. He used an albuterol nebulizer and inhaler last night with some relief, but today symptoms responded poorly to these treatments. Pt admits that symptoms feel similar to prior asthma exacerbations. He has been hospitalized for monitoring during acute asthma exacerbations in the past, but has no h/o acute respiratory distress or intubation due to this.

HPI #2: Janet Doe is a 32 year old female who presents with a persistent cough, dyspnea and fatigue for 1 week. She was seen here 3 weeks ago for rhinorrhea, nasal congestion and a sore throat, diagnosed as a viral URI after a rapid strep test was negative. These initial symptoms largely resolved 10 days ago, but then her present complaints began shortly afterward. She denies any fevers/chills. Admits to intermittent expectoration of clear and yellow sputum. Symptoms are improved with use of a home nebulizer and inhaler.

HPI #3: Johnny Doe is a 3 year old male who presents with a barky cough, shortness of breath and accessory muscle use while breathing. There are no apparent alleviating or exacerbating factors. His parents denied any evidence of a swallowed or inhaled foreign body. He is eating and drinking without obvious difficulty. The patient's older brother is currently ill with cold-like symptoms, but otherwise no known exposure to illness at daycare. Immunizations are up-to-date.

HPI #4: Little Sue is a 6 yo female who presents with a worsening episodic cough over the last week. The patient's cough becomes so severe at times that she vomits according to her mother. The episodes of coughing are increasing in frequency and the child seems to have problems catching her breath during them. Sue's sister is also starting to cough. The patient has not had a fever. The cough is not productive. Her mother states that she doesn't believe in vaccinations and the patient has therefore not received several of immunizations.

HPI #5: John Wilson is a 55 yo male who presents with dyspnea, productive cough, chest tightness and fever/chills. 5 days ago he developed a cough with clear sputum. Over the next 2 days this sputum turned green and he developed progressive dyspnea and chest tightness. This morning he spiked a fever and generally felt worse than the last few days, so he now presents for evaluation. Sputum is still green. Chest tightness is diffuse, pleuritic and worse with coughing. Denies hemoptysis.

HPI #6: Jane Doe is a 4 yo female who presents with a runny nose and cough for the last 5 days. Per mother, cough has been productive with clear sputum. Today, she spiked a fever of T max 100.7 F and has been fussier than usual.

Respiratory Answers

1. ***Asthma exacerbation.*** *This one is a gimme, because the patient has a significant history of asthma.*

2. ***Bronchitis.*** *A bronchitis is similar to pneumonia, though often lacks the chest tightness and colorful sputum of pneumonia. It can be defined quite simply as a productive cough without evidence of infiltrate (i.e. pneumonia) on a chest x-ray. Therefore, although this is much more suggestive of bronchitis, a chest x-ray will be necessary to differentiate between bronchitis and pneumonia.*

3. ***Croup.*** *This is a classic case of croup, which only occurs in young children and produces that pathognomonic barky cough.*

4. ***Pertussis (a.k.a. whooping cough).*** *This infection was largely quiet until the backlash against immunizations occurred sometime around 2010. Pertussis causes a very paroxysmal cough (described as episodic in the HPI) and the most important detail is that the mother has denied the patient from getting the usual vaccinations for her age.*

5. ***Pneumonia.*** *The key to this patient is the progression nature of symptoms that include green sputum and chest tightness.*

6. ***URI.*** *The key here is that the patient's cough produces clear sputum. The true differentiation of a URI vs a pneumonia will be the purpose of the workup, including a chest x-ray and labs.*

Hospital Notes: Discharge Summaries

EXAMPLE #1:

Principal Problem:

* UTI (urinary tract infection) due to yeast manifesting as altered mental status – treated with oral diflucan

Active Problems:

1. Acute renal failure – Cr 2.7, secondary to dehydration with elevated BUN:Cr ratio, improved with IV fluids
2. Unspecified essential hypertension
3. Restless legs syndrome (RLS) – at baseline
4. ACP (advance care planning) – full code
5. COPD (chronic obstructive pulmonary disease) – not an acute exacerbation
6. Anemia, unspecified, acute on chronic – status quo from prior admission, no transfusions

BRIEF HOSPITAL COURSE:

This 69 y.o. female who had a complicated hospital stay from 2/9/13-3/12/13 after a first round of chemotherapy for breast cancer that included emergent bowel resection and ostomy for ischemic colitis with uncontrolled bleeding, TPN, and profound weakness and malnutrition. She was treated with diflucan for a yeast infection in her urine revealed on a 3/4/13 urine culture.

She was discharged to a skilled nursing facility for therapy regarding her malnutrition and deconditioning, but returned 3/16/12 with renal failure, dehydration, and UTI. Again her urine culture demonstrated >100 K CFU of yeast. She is discharged back to SNF, and continued on a full course of 2 weeks diflucan. She should have a UA with culture in 2 weeks, and I also added nystatin powder in case she needs it. I also added a multivitamin (MVI) and iron supplementation to her program, and encouraged her to continue with good nutrition.

EXAMPLE #2:

PRINCIPAL DISCHARGE DIAGNOSIS: Acute gastroenteritis

Principal Problem:
*Acute gastroenteritis
Active Problems:
1. Atrial fibrillation
2. Major depression
3. S/P AVR (aortic valve replacement)
4. HTN (hypertension)
5. Chronic anticoagulation
6. Dementia
7. ACP (advance care planning)
8. Hip pain, left
9. Weakness generalized

BRIEF HOSPITAL COURSE:

This 88 y.o. male presented for evaluation of weakness, confusion, and diarrhea 3/19/13. PMHx significant for CAD, HTN, A Fib, CVA, prostate cancer, hyperlipidemia, anxiety, vertigo, hiatal hernia, and dementia. Recent admission 3/8 - 3/10/13 patient received antibiotics for UTI whose culture subsequently came back MRSA sensitive to nitrofurantoin. Clostridium difficile toxin negative. Stool culture negative. Likely simple ABX related diarrhea. Placed on metoprolol for rate control here and will halve dose at d/c given possible relation to AMS. He was agitated intermittently but less so at discharge. Paroxysmal asymptomatic afib while here with therapeutic INR on Coumadin. Patient has responded well to antibiotics but clearly deconditioned physically for which physical therapy has recommended subacute rehab.

EXAMPLE #3:

PRINCIPAL DISCHARGE DIAGNOSIS: Kidney stone on left side

Principal Problem:
 *Kidney stone on left side
Active Problems:
1. Mixed hyperlipidemia
2. Diabetes mellitus type II
3. Essential hypertension, benign
4. CME (cystoid macular edema)
5. BPH (benign prostatic hypertrophy)
6. GERD (gastroesophageal reflux disease)
7. COPD (chronic obstructive pulmonary disease)
8. ACP (advance care planning)

BRIEF HOSPITAL COURSE:

This obese 78 y.o. male has multiple medical problems including COPD, cystoid macular edema, benign prostatic hyperplasia, and GERD. He was admitted following a left ureteroscopy with laser lithotripsy, stone basketing. We were asked by urology to assist with medical management. Patient exhibited some fluid retention, was diuresed with Lasix, which he will discharge with as well. Patient was tolerating food well with no nausea on discharge. Has shown improvement from baseline in mobility, is encouraged to follow up with PT in outpatient. He was noted to desaturate with sleep suggesting obstructive sleep apnea. He will benefit from a sleep evaluation. No changes were made to the management of his other medical problems.

EXAMPLE #4:

PRINCIPAL DISCHARGE DIAGNOSIS: Accelerated hypertension

Principal Problem:
*Accelerated hypertension
Active Problems:
1. Hypertension – subsided with IV labetolol and started on 50 mg QD losartan
2. COPD (chronic obstructive pulmonary disease)
3. Hyperlipidemia
4. Chronic tension headaches
5. History of gastroesophageal reflux (GERD)
6. CKD (chronic kidney disease) stage 3, GFR 30-59 ml/min
7. N&V (nausea and vomiting)
8. FHH (familial hypocalciuric hypercalcemia)
9. Advance care planning
10. Anemia, chronic disease

BRIEF HOSPITAL COURSE:

This 74 y.o. female has a history of diabetes, hypertension, coronary artery disease, cerebrovascular disease and known tension headaches. She was admitted for evaluation of headache, nausea and vomiting in the setting of profound elevation of blood pressure - SBP at 220 on presentation. Negative head CT. She experienced a few loose stools following IV contrast for abdominal CT below. C.diff today was negative. Today she still complained of an occipital headache radiating to forehead. No fever or leukocytosis. BP is down following IV labetalol but still mildly elevated. Will keep her on losartan as outpatient until follow up with her PCP tomorrow for a blood pressure check.

Cardiology Consultation Note

REASON FOR CONSULTATION

49-year-old male who was admitted to hospital last week because of depression and chest pain. Referred here for follow up visit. No chest pain currently.

HISTORY

Pt has a long-standing history of depression with suicidal ideation and aggressive behavior. He has had several suicide gestures over the past 10 years. In addition, he has had intermittent chest pain going back several years. He tells me he had a negative stress echo at the University about a month ago. He was seen at Regency Hospital in February of this year with chest pain after using crack cocaine. Stress test was scheduled at that time, but was not done because he had eaten. It was thought that this was chest wall muscular pain. He has several risk factors. He is a smoker of 1-1/2 packs per day. He is obese. He has had borderline elevation of cholesterol. He has a very strong family history for heart disease. Both parents died of heart disease in their 60s. Several of his brothers have died at a young age of heart disease. There is also diabetes in his family.

PAST MEDICAL HISTORY

He had rotator cuff repair of the left shoulder.

HABITS

He drinks mostly on the weekends over a 6 pack. He denies crack cocaine for the past several months. His pain is pleuritic and there is tenderness in the chest wall.

REVIEW OF SYSTEMS

Otherwise negative.

SOCIAL HISTORY

He has worked as a laborer. He is married, and has no children.

MEDICATIONS

Lexapro.

ReVia.

Aspirin.

Nicotine patch.

Seroquel.

Trazodone.

PHYSICAL EXAMINATION

GENERAL: Pleasant overweight male in no acute distress, with somewhat flat affect.

VITAL SIGNS: Blood pressure 130/80, pulse 60 and regular, and temperature is normal.

HEENT: Head normal. Ears, nose, and throat negative.

LUNGS: Clear.

CARDIOVASCULAR: Heart normal. No murmurs, gallops, or rubs.

CHEST: There is chest tenderness over the lower lateral rib area.

GASTROINTESINAL: Abdomen is obese. No mass or tenderness.

EXTREMITIES: Normal.

LABORATORY DATA

Complete blood count was normal. Troponin negative x 2. ALT was 100. Other liver functions okay. Electrolytes okay. TSH was 0.27.

DIAGNOSTIC DATA

Electrocardiogram is normal x 2, and small Q waves in the inferior leads I suspect are normal.

ASSESSMENTS

1. Depression.

2. Alcohol abuse.

3. Tobacco abuse.

4. Chest pain, muscular.

5. Obesity.

PLAN

Reassure him that there is no evidence for heart disease, but he certainly needs to work on the risk factors. Follow up with primary physician to address these issues.

Ob/Gyn Clinic Progress Note

HPI: Jane Smith is a 37 y.o. female G3P2 female who presents for an annual gynecologic exam. She is doing well. She is not on the patch any longer. She had a saliva test done by her family's pharmacist in South Dakota. He told her that her estrogen levels were too high and that she needed some progesterone. She is now on these compounded creams and feels well. I warned her of the unproven benefits and risks of these creams. Please see ROS for any concerns.

MEDICATIONS:
- IBUPROFEN 200 MG TAB take 4 tablet (200mg) by oral route every 8 hours as needed with

ALLERGIES:
- Percocet (Oxycodone-acetaminophen) Itching
- Vicodin (Hydrocodone-acetaminophen) Itching

Past Medical History
- Endometriosis, Site Unspecified
  hyst

Past Surgical History
- Hx total abdominal hysterectomy 2006
- Hx salpingo-oophorectomy bilat

Social History
- Marital Status: Married

ROS:
GENERAL: She denies constitutional symptoms of fatigue, weakness, fevers, night sweats. SHE IS FRUSTRATED BY NOT BEING ABLE TO LOSE WEIGHT. HAS BEEN TO TWO WEIGHT LOSS SPECIALISTS AND THEY CAN'T FIGURE OUT WHAT IS WRONG. The remainder of the review of systems was completed and negative.

PHYSICAL EXAM:

Female who appears well and in no apparent distress. Alert and oriented x 3 BP 112/68 | Pulse 76 | Ht 1.651 m (5' 5") | Wt 80.287 kg (177 lb) | LMP Hysterectomy Body mass index is 29.45 kg/(m^2).

NECK: supple and free of adenopathy or masses

THYROID: normal without enlargement or nodules.

CHEST/HEART: Chest is clear, no wheezing or rales. No chest wall deformities or tenderness. Heart regular rate and rhythm normal S1 and S2, no murmurs

BREASTS: Symmetric, no dominant, discrete, fixed or suspicious masses are noted. No skin or nipple changes or axillary nodes. Self exam was discussed and encouraged.

GI: The abdomen is soft without tenderness, guarding, mass, rebound or organomegaly. Bowel sounds are normal. No evidence of hernias. WELL HEALED MIDLINE INCISION. HAD A RECENT BIOPSY TO THE LEFT OF THE MONS THAT WAS A PRECANCEROUS SKIN LESION.

GU: External genitalia, Bartholin's glands, Skene's glands, urethra and urethral glands are normal. Vagina has normal rugae and normal appearing discharge. Adnexa without masses or tenderness. Rectovaginal exam confirms bimanual exam and there are no unusual lesions or masses noted.

SKIN: only benign skin findings. No unusual rashes or suspicious skin lesions noted. Nails appear normal.

EXTREMITIES: Extremities: No clubbing, cyanosis, or edema.

MUSCULOSKELETAL: No obvious muscle atrophy. Patient able to move easily and capable of transferring to and from exam table autonomously. Able to lift arms easily for breast exam.

ASSESSMENT:

Encounter Diagnoses

• Dx: Routine Gynecological Examination Yes

PLAN:

Patient was given my handout on Routine Health Maintenance
Patient advised to return to clinic with any gynecologic concerns

INDEX

Zithromax, 200

Zosyn, 200

If you found the "Ultimate Medical Scribe Handbook, Primary Care: 3rd Edition" helpful and would like to take your education to the next level, Medical Scribe Training Systems offers a comprehensive online training course for primary care medical scribes. This course and our other courses are available for purchase year-round at www.MedicalScribeTraining.net. Each course is segmented into multiple modules based on a particular topic or topics. The organization of these largely follows the order found in this handbook but modules may include:

- Readings from The Ultimate Medical Scribe Handbook
- Video lectures
- Practice tutorials
- Supplemental handouts
- Flashcards and other activities
- Test(s)

Medical Scribe Training Systems is unique because of its discrete methodology to writing an eloquent history of present illness. Our courses will take the developing scribe through a step-by-step process, beginning first with simple practice HPIs that require little-to-no medical terminology, to more advanced HPIs that require knowledge of medications, medical terminology or labs (all elaborated upon within the course itself).

Courses are available for individual providers, physician groups, or medical scribe companies seeking to outsource scribe training. Visit us at MedicalScribeTraining.net to learn more about the national leader in medical scribe training or contact us directly at MedicalScribeTraining@gmail.com.

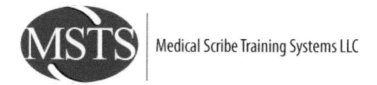
Medical Scribe Training Systems LLC

CPSIA information can be obtained at www.ICGtesting.com
Printed in the USA
LVOW01s0505150815

450250LV00034B/2362/P